Praise for Breathing Space

"I'm so grateful to have mindfulness resources like *Breathing Space for New Mothers* to recommend to my patients. As a reproductive psychiatrist, I'm always looking for ways to support women in their body-mind emotions and remind us all about the healing power of breath."

—ALEXANDRA SACKS, MD,
reproductive psychiatrist and author
of *What No One Tells You: A Guide
to Your Emotions from Pregnancy to
Motherhood*

"*Breathing Space for New Mothers* offers new mothers a mental shift—one that creates more room to trust ourselves, look after ourselves, and be ourselves even as we settle into this new role. It's a slowing down for our racing minds and our wild expectations, and it is truly a gift."

—KJ DELL'ANTONIA, author of
How to Be a Happier Parent and
former editor of the *New York Times*
"Motherlode" blog

"*Breathing Space for New Mothers* is not just a parenting guide, it's a life guide. This book is about cultivating a quality of being that allows us access to our deepest wisdom and intuition as mothers. Finally, a book that recognizes what is at the heart of parenting. The best thing we can do for our kids is be grounded and confident in our connection to ourselves and to them."

—HALA KHOURI, MA, cofounder
and director of Off the Mat into the
World and creator of the "Radiant
Pregnancy" online yoga video

Breathing
Space for
New Mothers

Breathing Space for New Mothers

Rest, Stretch, and Smile
One Yoga Minute at a Time

ALISON ROGERS WITH ERIN O. WHITE

North Atlantic Books
Berkeley, California

Published by   Cover design by Jess Morphew
North Atlantic Books   Book design by Happenstance Type-O-Rama
Berkeley, California   Illustrations by Yutaka Ai

Printed in the United States of America

Breathing Space for New Mothers: Rest, Stretch, and Smile—One Yoga Minute at a Time is sponsored and published by the Society for the Study of Native Arts and Sciences (dba North Atlantic Books), an educational nonprofit based in Berkeley, California, that collaborates with partners to develop cross-cultural perspectives, nurture holistic views of art, science, the humanities, and healing, and seed personal and global transformation by publishing work on the relationship of body, spirit, and nature.

North Atlantic Books' publications are available through most bookstores. For further information, visit our website at www.northatlanticbooks.com or call 800-733-3000.

MEDICAL DISCLAIMER: The following information is intended for general information purposes only. Individuals should always see their health care provider before administering any suggestions made in this book. Any application of the material set forth in the following pages is at the reader's discretion and is his or her sole responsibility.

Library of Congress Cataloging-in-Publication Data
Names: Rogers, Alison, 1952– author. | White, Erin O., author.
Title: Breathing space for new mothers : rest, stretch, and smile—one yoga
    minute at a time / Alison Rogers with Erin O. White.
Description: Berkeley, California : North Atlantic Books, 2019.
Identifiers: LCCN 2019017337 (print) | LCCN 2019020366 (ebook) | ISBN
    9781623173432 (E-Book) | ISBN 9781623173425 (paperback)
Subjects: LCSH: Motherhood. | Parenting. | Families. | Hatha yoga. |
    Self-actualization (Psychology) | BISAC: FAMILY & RELATIONSHIPS /
    Parenting / Motherhood. | HEALTH & FITNESS / Yoga. | BODY, MIND & SPIRIT /
    Meditation.
Classification: LCC HQ759 (ebook) | LCC HQ759 .R633 2019 (print) | DDC
    306.874/3—dc23
LC record available at https://lccn.loc.gov/2019017337

                    1 2 3 4 5 6 7 8 9 KPC 24 23 22 21 20 19

To Matt, Ted, and Nick,
the best of all teachers.

and

To all the women who manage to find grit
and grace in the midst of the messy, chaotic
love that is motherhood, may you—

"live like a river flows, carried by the sur-
prise of its own unfolding."

John O'Donohue

—AR

To my mother, Catherine White, who
found delight in motherhood and showed
me how to find it too.

—EOW

Contents

Introduction

Welcome

Do you remember the day you returned home with your baby? Maybe she was a few days old—or just a few hours. Perhaps your baby was born prematurely, and so your homecoming followed weeks of uncertainty and vigilance. Or maybe he was born in your bedroom, and your first journey was just a slow walk to the kitchen for a glass of water. No matter the circumstances, you traveled a great distance to an entirely new life. You stepped over the transom into motherhood, and chances are you are still acclimating to this undiscovered country. We want to welcome you. It's noisy and beautiful and wild, and we're so glad you're here.

As you read this, your baby might be sleeping or feeding, or maybe you are pushing a stroller with one hand and holding this book with the other. One thing we know for certain is that you've got a lot on your mind: vaccinations, diapers, feeding positions, laundry. And you're carrying a lot in your body too: healing incisions, swollen or even infected breasts, sore back, aching head. All this can make it nearly impossible to remember that you've recently been present at a miracle. Hell, you recently *wrought* a miracle! You made a baby. And because the experiences of birth and postpartum have such profound emotional and physical components, that miracle has changed you.

The answer to the equation baby+woman is not a simple one. Motherhood is a still-mysterious alchemy of hormones and experience and emotion that can't be easily teased apart. People talk about motherhood as a wild ride, or they talk about learning to surf the waves with your baby, but the truth is that you're not riding a wave, you *are* the wave, and you are being pulled toward the shore of your baby by the sheer force of her needs, which can't be delayed to a more convenient or relaxing time. Because what she needs is you.

Which is why it can be so easy to abandon yourself in these postpartum weeks and months. You might feel your needs pale in comparison to your baby's needs; you might feel selfish for thinking of what you need when there's this little helpless baby to take care of. And chances are you're not the only one whose attention is now entirely focused on the baby. You've traded a midwife or ob/gyn for a pediatrician, and no one is interested in your daily protein intake any more. It now takes significant effort to get the support you need, and so it can seem easier to just manage, to let things go and focus on the baby. "The baby is healthy—that's all that matters." We hear this all the time, in reference to everything from emergency C-sections to postpartum depression. But a healthy baby isn't all that matters. You matter. Because while it might feel wonderful to have the people you love care so much about your baby, there's no denying you could use a little care yourself. You are recovering from the strenuous physical work of labor and delivery. You need to take sitz baths or tend to a Cesarean incision, to feed yourself and mentally prepare for going to the bathroom. And as your baby gets older, you need to get some exercise or see a friend or get a little work done. You could use a whole team of supporting actresses to help you regain your strength and equilibrium. You could use some attention. You need to be seen and nurtured with compassion, even if everyone else in your world is entirely focused on the baby.

We want to pay attention to you so that you can bring some of *your own* attention back to yourself. In this book, every step of the way, we are thinking of *you* and how *you* are doing.

Breathing Space Is Not Just One More Thing . . .

The self-improvement industrial complex works hard trying to convince you that now is the time to enter into an intense postnatal campaign. Your pants size! Your pelvic floor! Your sex life! You've just had a baby, and suddenly the world is telling you just how much there is to fix. We don't think there's anything to fix, not your abs and not your attitude. We want to help soothe your tired mind and tired body, work with you to practice pausing every now and again to tend and befriend yourself, the self you are in this present—messy and imperfect—moment. *Breathing Space* is about doing something—very small and very quick—that feels good right away and that takes almost no time at all. Something you can do with your baby.

Breathing Space is about tuning in to your body and breath, but even more than that, it is about noticing sensations and feelings, getting to know yourself as a mother. In the first year of a child's life, her body and mind are changing at a rate that is never reached again, and is not seen in any other living creature. But *you* are changing too! This is a time of profound transition, one that has the potential for amazing self-discovery. But it's a real challenge for a mother to give herself the chance to reflect on her own experience, her own feelings. There is so much information about how to get to know your baby. There are tips on attuning to her, sensing her needs, learning to distinguish a hungry cry from a wet diaper cry. (Something that, by the way, even with five children between us, we were never able to do.) We're here to talk about finding yourself in motherhood so that you can grow into the mother you were meant to be, which is the only mother your baby needs.

Breathing Space is anti-advice. Advice has an odd way of making a new mother feel less capable, in the same way that just hearing the words "sleep while your baby sleeps" makes it nearly impossible to take a nap. We don't want to tell you what to do. There are more than enough books telling you how to be a better parent. It doesn't really matter if you use the Five S's, push your baby in a stroller, or carry her in a baby wrap. What matters is that what you are doing feels right for you and your baby. There are as many ways to raise a healthy child as there are cultures. In hunter-gatherer societies, three-year-olds wield machetes. In central Africa, the Efe women nurse each other's babies. All around the world, we see babies growing up to be competent and well adjusted in their communities. Research shows that your satisfaction—your sense of competence and pleasure—have a great impact on your child's sense of well-being. That satisfaction is what *Breathing Space* seeks to cultivate.

In early motherhood, when you're faced with a vast array of advice, ideas, methods, and practices, the first question to ask isn't, "What should I do?" The first question is, "What will work for my baby and me?" Finding the answer to that question can take some time and experimentation, and it starts with noticing how you feel in the moment and what your baby needs now. When you discover how strong, capable, and resourceful both you and your baby are, decisions become easier. When you are able to read your own signals and those of your baby with less worry and more realistic expectation, you can begin to know—and grow—your motherself.

But this takes a little while, and at first it's hard to figure out what your baby needs. When a friend of ours brought her two-week-old baby to the pediatrician with a list of questions, the doctor just smiled at her and said, "You're the one who knows this baby best. What do you think?" Our friend thought, *What?! I know her best? I hardly know her at all! This baby is screwed!*

While surely this pediatrician was trying to instill confidence in a new mother, his declaration had the opposite effect: panic. Getting to know your baby takes a while. But just because some things about him remain a mystery doesn't mean you aren't giving him just what he needs.

Until the Revolution

There are cultures in which postpartum mothers get attention and care, but contemporary American culture is not one of them. We live in a country with virtually no institutional support for new mothers. Paid maternity leaves are abysmally short (if offered at all), postnatal care is often perfunctory, and breastfeeding and childcare are seen as personal responsibilities rather than the public health and education issues they are. So we're going to deviate slightly from our anti-advice stance here, and gently suggest you *put down* any book about parenting—or close out any parenting website—that has the name of another culture in its title. French, Danish, German. Whatever—wherever—it is, whatever parenting method is being lauded, it's a parenting style that simply can't exist outside a country that sees the care of mothers and children as a collective responsibility. And in America we're not there yet. We've got a looong way to go.

There is so much work to be done. We want to be clear that *we know* there is work to be done. We know that it takes a village and that, chances are, you don't have one. And we know that if a woman lacks financial security, if she doesn't have a safe and comfortable home, a shift in perspective or the practice of mindfulness won't alter her circumstances. We don't subscribe to the idea that it doesn't matter what's happening, it's how you *think about* it. What's happening matters very much! We know that. And we know that many circumstances are stacked against even the most privileged American mothers, and that it can be nearly impossible not to internalize our culture's unbearably high expectations for you.

We also know that the more aware you are of what you feel and what you need, the easier it can be to ask for help. It's our great hope that mothers can begin to speak honestly with each other, their families, and their communities about their needs, and that such conversations can be a force for change, the beginning of a new way of talking about motherhood. We also know that it isn't your job to change institutions while caring for a baby. It is the responsibility of a civil society to create systems of care for mothers and babies that include generous parental leave and affordable, high-quality care and education for all children over one year of age. And we take that responsibility seriously.

New Mothers Are Wired to Love—and to Worry

It's not only unrealistic expectations that can make us feel anxious; new research tells us that our postpartum brains are wired for anxiety. In pregnancy and postpartum, brain activity increases in regions that control empathy, anxiety, and social interaction, and in this way, our brains orient us toward our babies, making it easier for a new mother to fall in love with her baby and also making us sensitive—perhaps overly so—to potential dangers. This increase in activity, coupled with a complicated cocktail of postpartum hormones, all predispose new mothers to be more emotional, attentive, and empathic.

In evolutionary terms, being hardwired for vigilance makes sense. But in the context of contemporary motherhood, it's more burdensome than lifesaving. Our babies are safe from the vast majority of threats that might have endangered our ancestors. We don't have to protect our babies from wild animals, plagues, or famine. But because our brains haven't caught up to these changes, we find new things to worry about. We chart sleep schedules and weight gain. We fret over progress toward developmental milestones; we cast sidelong glances at other mothers, convincing ourselves that they are doing it right, and we're not. We worry about brain development. We worry about allergies. We worry about swaddling and not swaddling. And when we're not worrying about something specific, we often feel a vague sense that something is wrong, with us or with our baby. This sense of unease is entirely understandable, for many reasons, chief among them the fact that new babies can be hard to read. A new father we know summed up the puzzle of newborn care perfectly when he said, "Who knew that the signs of perfect contentment and life-threatening dehydration are *exactly the same?*"

Because we are also experiencing such a profound increase in emotional openness, our feelings of love and attachment can leave us feeling raw, and our baby's vulnerability can seem nearly unbearable. So we become anxious. Who wouldn't? *Breathing Space* is about acknowledging and understanding that anxiety and gently training our minds and bodies to let it go. Because just noticing how often we are worrying—how often we think something is going wrong when nothing is actually going wrong—can be liberating.

Chronic anxiety—and its partner in crime, relentless self-criticism—are two of the biggest obstacles to enjoying motherhood. They drain available energy and distract you from your deeper feelings and from the present moment. And they drown out the voice of your nascent maternal instinct. When we talk about *maternal instinct,* we don't mean an innate sense of mastery or a preternatural knowledge of your baby. We are talking about a sense that you and your baby belong together, that you are a capable mother, and that your baby, even in his fussiest moments, is vigorous and well.

We have to learn to sort out unnecessary worry from helpful worry and to turn off unnecessary worry from time to time so we can rest and reset our own new and vigorous nervous systems. We need some breathing space. There are things you can do to settle the worry, although it will take some practice to get your postpartum mind on board, to gently remind your brain that no, the most relaxing use of your baby's naptime is not getting on the internet to confirm—yet again—that your jogging stroller isn't the model that was just recalled.

Practicing GRACE

The word *grace* means many things: elegance, finesse, agility, dignity, goodwill, generosity, kindness. A *grace period* is a time during which a demand is suspended, a debt forgiven. It is a respite and a reprieve.

Grace can also mean a blessing.

~~~

> *I do not understand the mystery of*
> *grace—only that it meets us where we are*
> *and does not leave us where it found us.*
> —ANNE LAMOTT

~~~

In *Breathing Space,* GRACE is an invitation to step out of the fray, to feel your feet on the ground, to relax tension in your body and mind. To reboot your hardworking nervous system.

GRACE is an acronym that guides you through a simple five-step exercise designed to create a clearing in body and mind.

♦ *Gather:* We gather and then shift our attention from the external busyness of life and our thinking mind to our body by focusing on the breath and our sensations, particularly the sensation of our feet solidly on the earth.

♦ *Rest:* On each exhale, we intentionally relax any tension in our jaw, shoulders, belly, and hands. We rest.

♦ *Ask:* We ask ourselves, "How am I feeling right now?" Then we allow whatever comes into awareness without resisting or arguing or shutting down.

♦ *Compassion:* No matter how we feel right now, how we are judging our self, we connect by remembering that mothers everywhere, throughout time, have felt the same things we are feeling. We treat our self like we would a dear friend—with understanding, attentiveness, curiosity, and respect.

♦ *Engage:* We engage life with our feet firmly planted on the ground in the present moment, our nervous system steadied and relaxed, and our heart softened, ready to begin again.

This ability to pause is so important right now. We know it can seem impossible. We know it might seem irrelevant. *We know the world is saying hurry up.* In the chaos of life with a baby whose needs are endless, who cares about your needs, your feelings?

We do.

Because we've been at this long enough to know that this motherhood gig just doesn't work unless you keep track of how you feel. Of how *you're* doing. Of what is working for you, and what isn't. Pausing, it turns out, is the single most important tool we have as mothers. Pausing is how we practice the art of recognizing that *this is not an emergency.* There will be emergencies, of course (and let us be the first to recommend you invest in a stack of navy-blue washcloths, as those tire-swing-to-the-nose trips to the emergency room go more smoothly when your child can't actually *see* the blood). But the emergencies will be infrequent. Mostly there will be decisions, chaos, conflict, desire, and disappointment. There will be children who refuse bedtime and baths, children who want piercings and skateboards, coed sleepovers and R-rated movies. And you'll need a moment to think of how you feel about it all. To think about what matters to you.

We repeat the five steps of GRACE in each of *Breathing Space's* ten practice sessions. Because the more you do it, the more empowering it becomes. And at some point, you will find yourself having a moment of GRACE in the heat of the moment, and you will feel grateful. For now, we just experiment and practice on the mat for a minute or two.

From Comparison to Kindness

The practice of GRACE cultivates self-compassion, which is the cornerstone of *Breathing Space.* Self-compassion reduces anxiety and the sense of isolation in mothers. Self-compassion is *not* self-pity. We've come to understand self-compassion as a kind of friendship with ourselves. From an early age, women are taught how to be good to our friends, to listen to their stories, to bolster their spirits in difficult times. To look at them with generous eyes. This is how we can see ourselves. We can be curious, loving, patient, impressed with all we have accomplished, excited by the great adventure of our lives.

At first it can be hard to see ourselves this way! But early motherhood is the perfect time to learn how. In this period, we have more capacity for love than at any other point in our lives. So why not include yourself in that expanding circle of love, protection, and care?

Sylvia Boorstein says, "let me greet the present moment as a friend," which seems like a great place to begin a practice of compassion. Because if you can greet this moment as a friend, you're greeting it with generosity and love. And by greeting it, you are, in a way, greeting yourself. Not the self that you were—or that you hope to be or wish to be or think you should be—but your present-moment self.

As mothers, we need connections, not comparisons. And we need compassion. The shift from a comparing mind to a kind mind is more important even than mindfulness. You can practice self-compassion by practicing GRACE. By pausing and resting long enough to ask yourself how you feel—and long enough to wait for an honest answer.

Kripalu Means Compassion

The seeds of *Breathing Space* were planted at Kripalu, a yoga retreat center in western Massachusetts where we—Alison and Erin—both attended retreats when our children were young. Those retreats were twenty years apart, and as different as night and day, but they changed us both in similar ways. Alison went to Kripalu first, when her first two sons were young. She left on a snowy morning in late spring, and still—to this day—remembers the sight of her husband and children standing at the window as she opened the car door to leave. The whole family had been sick with colds and was still recovering. She had planned her short getaway months before, her first since becoming a mother. Was she selfish? Abandoning her family? She was too worn out to answer those questions and too worn out to stay home. She got in the car and drove, hoping it was the right decision.

From the minute Alison walked through the doors of Kripalu, she knew it had been the right decision. The center was peaceful and bright, the people kind and caring. It was the perfect place to find some breathing space. Yoga at Kripalu was different; the teachers encouraged students to move slowly and to listen to their bodies with kindness and acceptance. She didn't know it at the time, but the word *kripalu* means "compassion." She left feeling deeply relaxed, more open, and patient with herself and her life.

It turned out that going to Kripalu for brief stays made her a better mother at home. So Alison returned to Kripalu again and again over the years. When her sons were grown, she earned her certification as a yoga teacher at Kripalu and began to dedicate herself professionally to the work of integrating psychology and yoga and mindfulness for new parents. As a result, Yoga of Parenting workshops and *Breathing Space* were born.

Erin also went to Kripalu in search of rest. And she also left her family—a wife and two daughters—with a hefty measure of ambivalence and guilt. But the purpose of her retreat wasn't to do yoga. It was to read a novel. That's right—she went to one of the country's most renown yoga and wellness retreat centers to read a book. Reading is how she makes sense of herself and the world, and it has been since she was a child. Books are her home. But since she'd had kids, Erin hadn't read much, and it was starting to feel like a piece of her—a very important piece—had gone missing. So Erin went to Kripalu and read a book. She read in the silent room and in the cafeteria. She read outside on the patio while the sun was setting. And by the end of the day—and the end of the novel—she felt like herself.

Like Alison, Erin didn't know that *kripalu* meant "compassion." And, like Alison, she was only just beginning to understand how to extend the same compassion she offered to her children to herself. Both Alison's and Erin's retreats allowed them—in different ways—to experience compassion in the literal sense of the word: they were "with" their own feelings of worry, desire, exhaustion, sadness, and love in a way that it wasn't possible to be with them at home.

Retreats are wonderful. But they can also be nearly impossible to arrange, for a host of financial and logistical reasons. Thankfully, you don't have to go away on retreat to learn to pause and relax. You can do it without leaving home or your baby. You can cultivate compassion right at home, right now.

Yoga Minutes

The "yoga minutes" you will find in this book reduce stress by focusing the mind on movement and breath. They increase flexibility and strength, and they help you to feel at home in your changing body. Yoga minutes give you a way to quickly and regularly check in with yourself in a calming and settling way. Each chapter of the book focuses on a theme and practice, then ends with a yoga minute, each one building on the next to create a ten-minute practice. But each practice also stands on its own, and you will find some that resonate with you and become your favorites for a while. You will become stronger and more resilient with each passing month, getting to know and accept your ever-changing, developing motherself and your baby.

Breathing Space Is for You

There are three different and short practices in each chapter: GRACE, breathing, and asana practice. Each practice can be done individually, but they also build on the previous chapter's practice, so that—when you have the time and energy—you can complete the book's full ten-minute practice. In this same way, you can dip in and out of the book at any time. It's all here for you.

Whether you have been practicing yoga and, like Alison, feel a disconnect between the yoga class and the practice of parenting, or if, like Erin, you are a person whose idea of yoga is a good stretch after a long nap, the practices of *Breathing Space* are for you. *And no matter how young or old your child is, is it is never too late to benefit from yoga and, in the process, improve your most important relationships.* Like a well-crafted yoga class, we begin with centering, move through warm-ups and postures, and we end with deep relaxation. At every step of the way, connections are made between yoga and parenting. The heart of yoga is compassionate awareness, the tools are breath and inquiry; it is rooted in the body. It is practiced with GRACE. Your mat is your safe haven for exploring and feeling and refining. There is no external ideal to match, no goal to achieve. We want you to make every breath, every pose your own. Modify the practices to meet your evolving needs. Now—take a slow deep breath and sigh it out.

Welcome.

Part One

MotherBaby

The Fourth Trimester

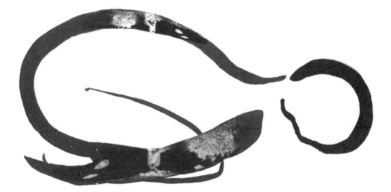

All this is to say that no matter how well you prepare for motherhood, you enter into it a changed person. You enter as a beginner, and you need to re-center, take breath, and figure it out.

Chapter 1

Coming Home

Maybe it was the underwear. Mesh boy shorts with a bright green stripe. Or maybe it was the pink plastic pitcher on the bedside table, which was making Abby shudder every time she looked at it. Why was a pink plastic pitcher of water making her shudder?

The thing was that the baby was absolutely fine, and so was she. There hadn't been any true emergencies, the close calls she'd heard about in her childbirth-preparation class. Thinking about that class now, it seemed hard to believe she'd ever gone to such a thing, ever sat on a floor pillow rubbing her stomach in a circle of other pregnant women also rubbing their stomachs, all listening attentively to a kind woman with a grey ponytail explain the difference between dilation and effacement. How had that even been her? First of all, Abby couldn't really sit anymore, and she sure couldn't sit on the floor. And the last thing she wanted to do was rub her belly, which, mysteriously, seemed to now be larger than it had been when she was actually pregnant.

Everyone was gone. "We want you to get some rest!" That's what everyone—the nurses, her husband, her visiting friends—had said. And they seemed so pleased that they'd made this rest possible. The baby was in the nursery; her husband had gone home to take a shower and walk the dog. "Now you can rest!" he'd said triumphantly before kissing her goodbye. "Okay, time for some rest!" the nurse had said, wheeling the baby out the room. And then that heavy, windowless door closed, and Abby was alone.

Get some rest? What did they mean? How, exactly, would Abby do that? Watch some television? Read a magazine? Just close her eyes and fall asleep? Every time Abby closed her eyes she saw the baby, felt that prickly sensation in her breasts, and then she *really* needed the baby.

She decided to give it a try. *I'll rest,* she thought. That's what the childbirth teacher had always said: "Sleep when your baby sleeps." It had seemed so logical then. Now it seemed like one of the stupidest things she'd every heard. But she was going to try.

She'd given birth right there, right there in that bed, in that room. It was something the hospital was proud of, that women didn't have to transfer to delivery rooms. But she wouldn't have minded a transfer. There was something about being in this very room, the room where nothing had gone wrong, not exactly, but also nothing had been exactly what she'd thought it would be. She'd expected pain, sure, but now she thought there should be a different word for what she'd felt. Pain was what happened when you broke your arm. This had been something else. This pain had an engine, a personality, it's own heartbeat.

Before the birth, Abby had thought she'd try all sorts of positions, the essential oil diffuser her sister sent her, and the playlist her husband had made. She'd hated all of it. She'd wanted total silence. She'd hated all the smells and hadn't wanted to be touched. She still felt terrible about that. All she'd wanted was to be totally still and focus entirely on the pink water pitcher. And then there'd been that moment of terrible fear, that one moment when everyone was telling her nothing was wrong—everything was fine—but they just needed a few minutes with the baby, just needed to check a few things before she could hold him.

And even though everything *was* fine, even though the baby wasn't gone for long, those were terrible, terrible minutes, and she didn't like thinking about them. She didn't like thinking about her beautiful baby being alone, without her.

Abby loved the baby. He was beautiful. He was like sunshine. That's what she would tell people when they asked what he looked like. *He looks like sunshine.* When he'd been taken out of the room—"Just for a moment! Everything's fine!"—the room was suddenly dark. The thought of that darkness gave her a stomachache.

Where was the baby right now, anyway? Was her resting time over? She was ready to be done resting. Should she push the call button? Maybe, but what would she say? She was embarrassed to say she didn't want to rest. *Sleep when the baby sleeps!*

Just then the windowless door swung open, and a nurse was there, holding a shrieking bundle of baby in her arms. "Well, someone's ready to eat," she said.

Relief! There was the baby. There was the sun. And also, that strange new prickly feeling in her breasts. The nurse handed Abby the baby. "Is Mom ready to feed?" she asked.

For an instant Abby was confused. She didn't know how to answer. Who was Mom? "Oh," she said suddenly realizing the nurse was referring to her, "you mean me!"

"Of course I do," the nurse said with a laugh. "Who else?"

"No one else," Abby said, trying to laugh a little too, even though it didn't seem that funny to her. No one else! No one else but her.

~ ~ ~

> I assure you
> There are many ways to have a child…
> There are many ways to be born.
> They all come forth
> in their own grace.
>
> —MURIEL RUKEYSER

~ ~ ~

You did it: you gave birth.

In a few short (although they may have felt very, very long!) hours of labor and delivery, your body has transformed, your identity has shifted, your hormones have gone into free fall, and people you don't even know are calling you Mom. It can feel like waiting for the navigation system to re-center, but it hasn't yet.

Now the baby you'd been waiting for is in your arms. You may be surprised at how madly in love you already are with her, and how protective you feel. Or you might not be feeling as in love as you thought you would. Or you might be in a strange in-between: crazy in love with a baby you don't know or understand at all. These early days with a new baby are all about that in-between.

When Alison was getting ready to go home with her first son, the nurses helped her dress and swaddle him, then Alison waddled over to dress herself, but between the huge episiotomy and the residual spinal block, she couldn't get her clothes on. So the nurse helped her get dressed too. The nurse then put Alison and her baby in a wheelchair and wheeled them out of the hospital to a car driven by her husband, who also had no clue how to take care of a baby. As they drove away, Alison looked back longingly at the hospital with all its help and support. She looked at her husband and then at the baby in that huge car seat, and she thought there had been some mistake.

But there was no mistake; there was just the *in-between,* that unsettling, entirely unknown territory between the hours of birth and the weeks (and months) of becoming a mother. The nurse, the pediatrician, the woman at the grocery store check out—they might all call you Mom, but that doesn't mean you feel like one. And it doesn't mean you should. You can still call yourself by your name.

And You Can Begin to Tell Your Story

Chances are your birth experience is a powerful memory, a visceral feeling. But it might not be a story quite yet. Or, at least, it's not the story it will become, as you recollect all the moments of amazement, confusion, fear, laughter, and pride, and blend them with the recollections of the people who were there with you. We encourage you to talk about your birth as much as you want, as much as you are able. Don't worry about repeating yourself! Tell your partner, your family, your friends, and, by all means, tell you baby. The poet Muriel Rukeyser said the universe isn't made of atoms; it's made of stories. We think this is true of babies and mothers too. We are made of stories. And in a world that doesn't always listen so closely to the stories of women's lives, it's important to know that your birth story matters.

It's also important to know that it's an extraordinary, heroic story even if it's not the story you were expecting to tell, even if your birth didn't go the way you imagined it would. In truth, *no* birth goes the way a pregnant woman imagines it will, because birth is, by its very nature, unpredictable. We live in a world in which our watch can tell us how many hours we spent in REM sleep, but still no one—not a doctor, fortune teller, mystic, midwife, or robot—can tell us exactly what a birth is going to be like.

Giving birth in the United States at this particular moment in time means that many of the details and logistics of your birth will be as expected, but each birth is still as original as the baby it brings into the world. Having a baby means taking part in one of our world's last true mysteries, our last unknowns. You entered it, you experienced it, and now you are on the other side. *You did it.*

Great Expectations

Even when we acknowledge the mystery and the unknown of it all, we can be caught off guard when the expectation and the reality of birth are so far apart. And sometimes that disconnect can make us do strange things. When Erin was in labor with her first baby, she didn't go to the hospital until she was nine centimeters dilated, because all during her pregnancy she'd been thinking about how much pain there would be during labor, and when the actual labor pain was really intense (so intense!) she still thought, *Well, this is bad, but I* know *it's going to get a lot worse.* Turns out that she actually *didn't* know that. She didn't know anything. All she had were her expectations. And because her expectations and her reality were entirely out of alignment, she almost gave birth in a parking lot.

Abby, too, was caught off guard when her expectation and her reality didn't match up. And this disconnect left her shuddering at the sight of a pink hospital pitcher. You might also be having a visceral response of some kind when you think about your birth. Maybe, like Abby, you experienced an unexpected separation from your baby after the birth. Perhaps you were expecting to give birth without an epidural, and you ended up asking for one. Or you were hoping for an epidural, and there wasn't time. Our contemporary culture places significant emphasis on planning for birth, and because of this, during pregnancy, we are as ripe with expectations as we are with baby. All this can leave us feeling let down by our birth experience, or—perhaps worse—that we've let someone down.

You haven't let anyone down.

You gave birth. You brought a baby into the world. You entered into a physical and emotional unknown that no one could entirely prepare you for or thoroughly explain. You met the uncertainty; you faced the pain. You may have been scared, but you did it all anyway.

You did it.

This is an important thing to remember. So important, in fact, that it's our book's first mantra. *I did it.*

We love mantras. We find that they help us focus, help us calm down, help us "fake it until we make it." Although "fake it" isn't really what we want to say. You're not faking it. You are doing it. So maybe a better way of saying this is that mantras help us "speak it until we mean it."

A mantra can help your mind catch up with a new reality, and in the case of the first postpartum weeks, there is a lot of catching up to do. It can take a while, much longer that the six weeks until your postnatal checkup, much longer than the twelve weeks until the end of the "fourth trimester," that relatively new term for the three months following birth when the baby is getting accustomed to the world outside the womb and the mother is getting accustomed to, well, everything.

Babies Have a Loose Relationship with Time (Which Means, Unfortunately, That Now You Do Too)

One of the hardest, most absurd things to get used to is your new relationship with time. Or perhaps it's not a relationship so much as it is a breakup. You can no longer rely on two in the morning to be what it once was: a time you saw on the clock when you were closing down the bar with friends or suffering from a bout of insomnia. Whatever the reason you were up then, and however frustrating it might have been to be awake in the night, chances are no one needed anything from you in those midnight hours. You could lie in bed quietly or read or watch infomercials. But now, when you're awake in the night, someone most definitely needs you. Two in the morning might as well be two in the afternoon as far as your new baby is concerned. At two in the morning, you might be feeding, changing diapers, dancing around the house with a screaming baby, or eating pretzels and reading the news on your phone while your baby happily kicks and gurgles on the changing table. It's a terribly disorienting shift in time. And it can be unsettling, even frightening.

When Erin's first child was a newborn, Erin lived in fear of the evening hours. Every afternoon at five she began to feel a terrible panic set in, the feeling that she wouldn't make it through the night. Some of this panic, this anxiety, was because she was exhausted and didn't know what the night had in store for her. But some of this anxiety—a great deal of it, actually—was biological. Although Erin didn't understand this at the time, her brain had actually changed during pregnancy, adapting to make her more sensitive to threats to her baby's safety, threats like the onset of darkness, the beginning of evening. Because even though we humans are long past the time, evolutionarily speaking, when we needed to protect our babies from nocturnal predators, our brains haven't quite caught up to our modern existence. A new mother's brain is still wired for worry and for vigilance. We'll explain those brain changes in more detail in chapters to come, but for now we'll focus on where that worry and vigilance plays out: your nervous system.

Did You Know …

Your nervous system is made up of two parts, sympathetic and para-sympathetic, and they each do different things in the body. The sympathetic nervous system is the first line of response to perceived threat or stress, specializing in fight-or-flight reactions. It makes your heart beat faster and stronger, opens your airways so you can breathe more easily, and inhibits digestion (in order to shift all available blood flow to more important bodily functions). These are all helpful if you are in danger or if your baby is in danger. It helps you to react quickly and efficiently.

The parasympathetic nervous system, on the other hand, is responsible for bodily functions when we are relaxed or at rest: it stimulates digestion and helps us to relax. It is sometimes called the rest-and-connect response.

In early postpartum, it can be difficult to shift gears from the high alert of the sympathetic response to rest-and-connect of the parasympathetic response. And that's where yoga comes in.

Yoga is sweet relief and rest. Mindful yoga, with its emphasis on movement and slow, deep breathing, has been shown to effectively shift the nervous system into the safe mode. It is the perfect antidote for new mothers. Yoga has been shown to decrease stress hormones and inflammation and to increase the body's neurotransmitters that are associated with relaxation. As your nervous system is soothed and calmed, you can be more present and less reactive. You can feel a bit of space open up, giving you the freedom to pause and choose a response, rather than react automatically in a rigid, anxious way.

Your baby gives you feedback about what he needs and likes. In the same way, your body will give you feedback about what *you* need and want. But it's hard to hear your body's messages when your nervous system is stressed. Stress leaves your nervous system with pretty limited options for response: fight, flight, or freeze.

In order to free our bodies and minds to respond in more open and varied ways, we have to relax and nourish the nervous system. And while this can sound complicated (or even impossible), it's not. We relax the nervous system by pausing. By pausing and by bringing our attention to our breath and to our body. Yoga is a reunion, a time to reunite your body, heart, and mind—all three evolving—through breath and movement. It is a way for you to create breathing space.

One Minute Yoga 1

A New Kind of Rest: GRACE

But before we begin yoga, we pause. We pause to stop what we are doing for just a few seconds and come home to our body and our breath. In this pause we learn to pay attention with kindness.

Knowing all that you have just gone through, we want to give you ways to rest briefly—and often. A way to switch your nervous system to safe and relaxed. In this practice, you engage your mind just enough to relax your nervous system. You can do it for just a minute, anytime you need it. The more you do it, the better it feels.

GRACE 1

- *Gather* your attention inward by feeling your body touching the bed that is holding you.

- *Rest* your jaw and shoulders; let your body sink into the bed.

- *Ask* "How does my body feel right now?" "Where is there discomfort; where is there comfort?"

- *Compassionately,* and with great kindness, acknowledge all that you have been through and send loving breath to any places that hurt.

- *Engage* life as it is now, feeling grateful for all that you did to birth your baby. Begin again.

Breathing 1

Find any position that is comfortable. At first you will probably want to be lying down, with pillows as needed. Later, if you want, you can try child's pose or practice while feeding your baby. This time and space will become your refuge, a small retreat that you can count on each day. You can play soothing music or pause in silence.

How about trying it right now? First just notice how your body feels on the bed. Observe how you can let go and be held by the safety of the surface. Place one hand or a pillow on your belly, the other hand on your heart. Simply follow your breath with your attention.

Now, lengthen and deepen both the inhale and exhale to the count of four. Feel belly, ribcage, then chest expand on the inhale. It's important to relax your belly as you inhale. Notice your chest, ribcage, and then belly contract on the exhale. This is called three-part breathing *(dirga pranayama)*. If your mind wanders, don't worry—that's what minds do. Just bring your attention back to your breath. If you need a stronger breathing pattern, you can try what is aptly called "victorious breath" *(ujjayi pranayama)* or "ocean-sounding breath." Breathing through your nose, press the back of your tongue gently up to the roof of your mouth so that your breath sounds like the waves of an ocean for a count of four. Victorious breath requires a little more effort, which can be more energizing and can engage your attention more. Try three rounds of breath—either three-part breathing or victorious breath.

Asana 1

YOGA REST

For this first month, there is no special posture or movement; we are simply learning the art of paying attention to and relaxing our physical body. Bring your attention to the top of your head and relax any tension you feel there, and then shift your attention slowly down your body, relaxing and releasing tension from each part, one by one: your forehead, your jaw, your shoulders, arms, chest, belly, pelvic area, legs, and feet. Finish by taking three more slow breaths and add your mantra to each breath: think *I* on the inhale and *did it* on the exhale.

For the next few weeks you will be feeding, changing diapers, making it through another night of less sleep. You can breathe deeply and acknowledge all of these accomplishments with this one-minute yoga.

Mantra 1: I did it.

Chapter 2

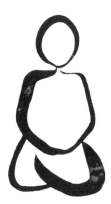

Easy Pose

In the weeks following her daughter's birth, Dana liked to imagine her living room as the set for a play. Never before had it contained so many *things*. A bassinette, a swing, an infant seat, a brochure about banking cord blood (they hadn't done it, a decision which Dana already regretted), a damp nursing bra, a baby monitor that was always on and hissing, even when the baby was right next to her. And today there she was, the star of her imaginary show, her shirt open, a breast pump and two bottles of milk on the coffee table next to her, typing on her phone. Working. On what was supposedly her maternity leave.

Dana wished her old, pre-baby self could see her now, that opinionated and well-rested woman who would never have let a baby take over her life, and certainly not her living room. She'd refused a baby shower, insistent that all a baby needed was a stack of diapers and a place to sleep. Three weeks in, and Dana had ordered two showers' worth of baby paraphernalia, delivered by a UPS man who came so often he was like family.

What were you thinking? Dana silently asked her old and entirely foreign self. *Who were you?*

As if following a stage direction, Dana's mother came into the room. "Hon, why don't you take a walk while she's still sleeping?"

Dana put down her phone. "I was going to give her a bath."

"I can do that when she wakes up."

"Oh, that's okay, Mom," Dana said. Suddenly Dana's play was taking a dark turn, a wet baby slipping through the hands of a frail and elderly woman. Never mind that Dana's mom wasn't even sixty and did Pilates three times a week.

"No, really, you should go," her mother insisted. "I know how to bathe a baby, for god's sake. Go out and feel the sun and see the trees. Go!"

Dana was too tired to object. And, she had to admit, she was desperate to get out of the house alone. She closed her shirt, made her slow way up from the couch cushions to find her shoes and her husband's jacket. "When will I be able to close my own jacket?" she asked.

"It's only been three weeks," her mother said. "They say nine months on, nine months off."

"Yeah, well, they also say a good birth plan prevents an unnecessary C-section."

"You inherited Nana's small hips. Let's blame her."

"You blame her for everything. Is Mabel going to blame me for everything?" Dana's mother opened the front door and gently pushed Dana onto the porch.

"Probably. But you've got some time," she said. "Enjoy it while you can."

Here's something else Dana hadn't expected: when she was with the baby, she wanted to take a break from her. And when she got a break, she wanted to be with the baby. All her long-loved pleasures—a night in a hotel, a long hike with a friend, a swim in the ocean—were things she both desired beyond reason and never wanted to do again. Because now there was a baby in the world who was hers, and even if she were away from her, she was never out of her mind. The guilt, the guilt. Her whole life, people had talked about mothers and their guilt, and Dana had wondered what the big deal was. Now she knew. She knew, and it was crushing. It made contentment, the simple enjoyment of a solitary moment, entirely impossible.

Although now she was feeling okay; she was feeling fine. She decided to walk a little further, maybe even do a lap around the park. It was nice to be out—her mother was right. She passed some construction, with a bright orange-and-black detour sign, which reminded Dana of all the signs in the delivery room. All the beeping. And the doctor's voice, which was too serious, too urgent, saying words like *decels* and *meconium.*

She thought that birth would be a crazy and wild ride, a great story, but instead hers had been a series of close calls and narrow escapes, a story she didn't want to tell but couldn't get out of her mind. And now she remembered something else, something about how babies can drown in an inch of water. Or was it half an inch? She immediately turned around and started for home, moving in a sort of hobbling waddle-jog, the fastest pace that her aching C-section incision would allow. This would not, she told herself, be a scene in the play.

Dana rushed into the house. Her mother was standing in the living room with the baby, who was wrapped in a towel and shrieking, a shock of wet black hair plastered against her little head. "She's been fine," Dana's mother said, a bit defensively. "You didn't need to rush."

Dana took the baby from her mother's arms, sat down on the couch. The baby quieted. Dana lay her head back against the pillows and closed her eyes. She kicked off her shoes. She took a slow breath, and another. She smelled the baby's head. Dana's mom sat down next to her, holding a magazine. "This one has a quiz," Dana's mother said gently. "Want me to read you the questions?"

Dana loved magazine quizzes, as did her mother and her grandmother. She'd been raised on them, and she'd long loved how answers to trivial questions allowed for grand and illuminating classifications of a self. But she hadn't wanted to do one since the baby was born. She'd like to say that it all just seemed silly, but honestly, more than that, it just seemed sad. She was entirely unclassifiable. She was a mystery.

"We could answer for the baby," her mother suggested. "Instruct her in the ways of our people."

Dana laughed, which, like so many things now, both made her incision ache and made her feel better. She held the baby aloft, letting the towel fall onto her lap, and she marveled at the baby's tiny perfect nakedness. "Okay, Mabel," she said. "Let's get started. Let's find out who you are."

~ ~ ~

This is hard. Relax. Take a Breath. Let's
pay attention to what is happening. Then
we'll figure out what to do.

—SYLVIA BOORSTEIN

~ ~ ~

A baby changes everything.

Your body, your hormones, your emotions, your living room. And, as we talked about in chapter 1, pregnancy changes your brain. Researchers have recently discovered pregnancy and early motherhood cause long-term changes to brain structure. When researchers from Europe and the United States compared the brain scans of new mothers to those of women who'd never been pregnant, they found significant differences between the two. The brain scans of new mothers showed alterations in the area of the brain responsible for social processing—in particular, the capacity to accurately read facial expressions and experience empathy. The researchers suggest that these pregnancy-induced brain changes, which last for at least two years, are caused by hormones and are an evolutionary development that prepares a mother's brain to care for a baby.

Researchers see changes in brain areas responsible for caretaking, motivation, and reward, and—here's the tricky part—in areas associated with obsessive anxiety. This means that a mother's brain is wired for love, sensitivity, and bonding, but that this love and impulse for connection are neurologically tangled up with worry. This means that new mothers can easily, and understandably, become obsessed with worries.

On top of all this, new mothers experience profound relational changes. You are becoming a mother at the same moment your parents are becoming grandparents. And your partner, who until recently was a friend and a lover, is now your co-parent. The person whom you must negotiate and collaborate with in the care of the being you both love most. And you used to think it was hard to pack the trunk together!

All this is to say that no matter how well you prepare for motherhood, you enter into it a changed person. You enter as a beginner, and you need to re-center, take a breath, and figure it out. There's just no way around it! You're a beginner at something you've been told comes naturally, as though motherhood were a reflex or maybe a universal developmental stage, like puberty. As wonderful as it can feel to love a new baby so deeply, so astonishingly, motherhood is a role and a job that doesn't come naturally to most of us. But what *can* seem to come naturally is insecurity and self-doubt.

Maybe all we want is time alone with our baby, but our mother, friend, or partner swoops in to help by taking our baby and shooing us out for fresh air. We want to feel grateful, but we feel displaced and uneasy. Or maybe we don't have enough help, and all we want is a break from our baby, and we feel guilty about that. All this is perfectly normal. Not pleasant, but normal. Every bit as normal as the mistakes you will inevitably make. We—all parents—make so many mistakes! With five children between us—Alison and Erin—spanning multiple eras of child-rearing advice and norms, we've made pretty much any mistake you can think of. We've forgotten to buckle the baby into the car seat. We've left the house without diapers and wrapped our favorite scarf around our baby's butt. We've put babies in a bath that was too cold, and we've dressed them too warmly for bed, then found them so slicked with sweat you'd think they'd snuck out for a jog. We've given them so much rice cereal they didn't poop for a week. We've put off going to the doctor when it turned out to be strep; we've gone to the ER when it turned out to be gas. And why wouldn't we make mistakes? No one would expect us to sit down at the piano for the first time and play a concerto perfectly.

We're Absolute Beginners….

Remember that David Bowie song, the one about soaring over mountains with nothing to lose? Well, being an absolute beginner at motherhood is a little bit like that, except you probably feel you have everything to lose. Which means that you have to be brave. It means failing and trying again. It means taking a breath, then figuring it out.

You might be thinking, *Easy for you to say! I've got a fragile-looking human being here. My human being! I don't have time to breathe!* And you're right. There is so, so much at stake with a baby. But you do have time to breathe. Because moment to moment, day to day, you *are* doing this. You are feeding, diapering, rocking, soothing, bathing. You may feel anxious or exhausted or worried, but that doesn't mean you aren't handling the essential tasks of motherhood. That doesn't mean you aren't taking wonderfully good care of your baby. You can take a breath and figure it out. There's time for a breath. There's time to figure it out. You are doing this.

The transition to motherhood offers endless opportunities for harsh self-judgment. But the opportunities for growth and a new and profound form of love are just as endless. Love for your baby, but also love for your imperfect self, your imperfect life.

For some of us, self-compassion is a new concept, but there is no time like the transition into motherhood to learn the skills of self-compassion. We can learn to be as gentle with our new motherself as we are with our new baby. Self-compassion makes it easier to have compassion for your own parents, partner, friends, and colleagues.

~ ~ ~

> *Compassion is aimed at the alleviation of*
> *suffering—that of others or ourselves—*
> *and can be ferocious as well as tender.*
> —KRISTIN NEFF

Did You Know …

Self-compassion is associated with emotional resilience. Research shows that the more self-compassionate a person is, the less likely she will suffer from anxiety or depression. But what is self-compassion, and how is it different from self-esteem and self-pity? Self-esteem is contingent on perceiving yourself as successful at meeting goals. *I feel good about myself because I was able to soothe my baby.* The problem with self-esteem is that because it is contingent on meeting expectations, when we *aren't* able to soothe our baby, we feel like we have failed and often then we judge ourselves harshly. On the other hand, self-compassion is not contingent on success or judging ourselves or comparing ourselves favorably to others.

Self-compassion is different from self-pity. Self-pity is often expressed as a question: *Why me? Why does my baby have colic and cry for hours?* It leads to feeling powerless and isolated. Self-compassion, on the other hand, is an acknowledgement, *I am doing everything I know how to do to soothe my baby, and still she is fussy. Like all the other mothers who have babies who are hard to soothe, I need some kindness and some help.*

Kristin Neff, a pioneer in the field of self-compassion research, defines self-compassion as "a way of relating to ourselves kindly as we are in this moment, and embracing ourselves, as we are, flaws and all." According to Neff, there are three core components of self-compassion. First is the awareness of how we are feeling. This can be difficult in the moment, but it gets easier with practice. Second is the recognition that we are not alone. We can take a moment to realize that all mothers everywhere, at times, feeling unsure, make mistakes, and try again. The third component is treating ourselves with kindness. In those tough times when things aren't going well or when you make a mistake, you can try to talk to yourself the way you would a dear friend, with patience, sympathy, and gentleness. You might say to yourself, *I am feeling worried so much of the time, and while I know that there are other mothers who are experiencing this same thing and that I am not alone, this is still so hard. I will be kind to myself—it will get better.* You can say to yourself, *Take a breath, then you'll figure it out.* When you practice self-compassion instead of self-criticism, you practice self-soothing, kindness, and curiosity. The result is problem solving and empowerment rather than self-pity or self-blame.

Mindful yoga is a physical expression of self-compassion. We offer compassion to our body, mind, and heart by giving it some loving attention through stretching, soothing, and opening. Yoga moves us out of our heads and into our bodies by yoking the breath with movement and focusing attention on the body and its sensations rather than the thinking mind. Yoga gives you the tools to relax and reset your nervous system. As the nervous system relaxes, it becomes easier to pay attention with gentle compassion toward yourself.

But before we practice yoga we have to stop doing everything else. We might only need to stop for a moment, but we do have to stop. And stopping is hard! Preparation rituals can help. Remember the moments before the beginning of a group class at a yoga studio? You enter the studio, take off your shoes, get your props, arrange your props, choose two blocks, go back to get two different blocks, see the blanket of the person next to you, which is clearly softer than yours and causes you to debate for a moment going back and getting a better one. You forget your strap, go back for a strap, wonder if you'll need a strap at all, and hope you don't, because honestly you don't love using the strap—you can never get the buckle quite right. You wish for a moment that you'd worn different yoga pants—where were those other yoga pants anyway? You wish you'd brought a hair tie, wish you'd taken out your earrings. But then, no matter what, class begins and you have to stop. You have to pause all the movement and rumination and longing so that you can begin.

At home, in daily life with a baby, you can still give yourself ample opportunities for a preparation ritual, because it can be even harder to stop in a place where there are so many other things to do. To prepare at home you can take a few minutes to arrange a space, maybe push the coffee table over a few inches to make way for a cushion or mat or move the laundry to the other side of the bed. You can put on socks or take them off, drink a glass of water, realize you're too hungry to begin and eat a peanut butter sandwich. All these preparations are fine. Go ahead and do any of them. Or do all of them! And when you're done, and there's nothing left to do, lie down on your back or rest in child's pose. Or sit up on a blanket, block, or cushion. Put your baby down, or pick him up and settle him in your arms.

After a bit of practice, you might not need to do any of these things before you begin. Or maybe you will. Either way, just do them, and then finish doing them. And then stop, so that you can begin.

Sometimes it helps to have a small physical reminder around the house, something that will cue you to take a moment for yourself. It could be a photograph, a mala bead bracelet you wear, a piece of pottery, a postcard, or a few lines from a favorite poem or song. Anything that can catch your eye and remind you to pause for a moment.

One Minute Yoga 2

GRACE 2

- ♦ *Gather* your attention by looking at your environment and name three things you see. Then feel your body touching the ground, seat, or bed.

- ♦ *Rest* by feeling your breath as it enters and exits your nostrils. Now notice how your belly feels as you breathe, *relax* your belly on the inhale, instead of "holding it in." Bring some love to that belly.

+ *Ask* "How am I talking to myself, right now?" "Can I be kinder, right now?"

+ *Compassionately* allow that you may be self-critical—it's what our minds do. It is our attempt at self-improvement.

+ *Engage* again with your day feeling softer and kinder toward yourself—belly, mistakes, and all. Begin again.

Breathing 2

ALTERNATE-NOSTRIL BREATHING

This month the breathing practice is alternate-nostril breathing *(nadi shodhana)*. It's an excellent, effective way to calm and balance the nervous system quickly.

In a comfortable seated position or lying down, take one slow, deep breath in and out.

Raise the thumb and ring finger of your left hand to your nose.

(Note: if you are breastfeeding, use whatever hand is free.)

On the next breath, close off your right nostril with the ring finger and breathe in through your left nostril to the count of three or four.

Close both nostrils for one to two seconds, or longer, if it's comfortable, while you hold in your breath.

Open your right nostril and exhale.

Hold with both nostrils closed.

Open the right nostril and breathe in.

Hold both closed.

Exhale out the left side.

Repeat alternating sides with a steady breath for thirty seconds or so.

End with a full inhale and exhale through both nostrils. Close your eyes and feel the effects of the breathing practice. Notice any changes.

Asana 2

+ Sit in a comfortable way on a blanket or cushion on your mat, or on your bed or chair for easy pose.

+ Inhale slowly and raise both arms out to the sides, to shoulder height, palms facing forward.

+ Exhale as you round your back and gently hug yourself.

+ Inhale as you open your arms until they are behind you and your back is arched, and lift your chest, and then lift your chin slightly.

+ Exhale and round your back and hug yourself again.

+ Repeat three times. See if you can make the movement and breath rhythmic and slow.

Mantra 2: Take a breath, then we'll figure it out.

Chapter 3

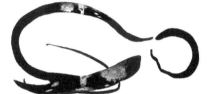

Child's Pose

"Well, good night," Melanie said, pausing at the bedroom door after she'd finished brushing her teeth. Her husband, Joe, was already in bed.

"Good night," he said, leaning over to turn out the light. "And good luck."

At first, it had seemed funny, this thing that they said to each other every night before one of them went to sleep in their bed and the other went into the living room to bounce, cajole, sing, hum, and chant their newborn baby into a maddeningly brief few hours of sleep. In the beginning, this arrangement had seemed manageable, but now that Joe was back to work, he only did a few shifts a week. Most nights it was Melanie, who was still on maternity leave. And "the beginning" was starting to seem like a long time ago. The baby was almost three months old, which meant it had been almost three months since Melanie and Joe had slept in the same bed. But this was what it took to keep the baby happy and, more importantly, quiet.

Melanie and Joe lived in an apartment building, with neighbors on every side. In the first two weeks of the baby's life, they made daily batches of "Sorry about the Crying!" cookies. Everyone had been pretty nice about it, but Melanie had lived in apartment buildings most of her life, and she knew that the sound of a crying baby could get very annoying, very fast. So it was important that the baby, once it was nighttime, not cry. This wasn't easy. This baby was a real crier. What they'd discovered, about a week after they'd come home from the hospital, was that the only way he'd sleep was when he was actually on someone's body. In the beginning this was okay. Her husband was off work for a week, and then Melanie's mom came for a few days. They all traded off, and that was nice. It worked. But that was a long time ago now. Her mom had gone home, and her husband had been back at work for months. And this was what they'd figured out: Melanie would sleep on the couch, with the baby in a Bjorn.

They'd tried everything. And this was what worked: she fed the baby in very small doses, always burped him, and never put him horizontal for the first half hour after a feeding. The doctor had suggested a swing, but he hadn't liked it, and they really had too small of an apartment to use something that took up that much space. After a week they'd put it on Craigslist.

"Babies cry," said her mother-in-law, who had raised her own babies on a farm in upstate New York, with only the horses and chickens to bother. "You can't let it upset you so much."

But it did upset Melanie, and not just because of the neighbors. She wanted some quiet too. She wanted to stop living this way. She wanted—and was this too much to ask?—to just sleep, for one night, next to her husband in her own bed.

~ ~ ~

> *Yoga teaches us to cure what need not*
> *be endured and endure what cannot*
> *be cured.*
>
> —B. K. S. IYENGAR

~ ~ ~

Are you doing something that is starting to feel crazy and unsustainable? It could be nursing a baby every two hours around the clock or driving around town to get your baby to fall asleep, only to have her wake up as soon as you bring her into the house. Or maybe you've given up on bringing her into the house, so, like Audrey and Jeremy in "The Letdown," you're having sex in the car, because it's the only place the baby will stay asleep—that is, if you're having sex at all. And maybe, right about now, it feels like things are never going to change, like you'll be driving and soothing and swaddling this tiny baby forever. But you won't. Right about now it's so important to remind yourself that *it's temporary.*

Alison studied anthropology in graduate school and decided she would soothe her third baby the way hunter-gatherers did: by keeping him in physical contact with her all the time. What she'd forgotten was that those hunter-gatherers she'd once studied live communally, with lots of "alloparents": relatives, friends, and neighbors who share in the care of the young. No mother is isolated and in constant physical contact with her child. Not surprisingly, Alison's cross-cultural approach to infant care was exhausting. And, also not surprisingly, her son became accustomed to on-demand night nursings that lasted more than a year.

Accumulated sleep deprivation and crying are the hallmarks of the third month of motherhood. We exhaust ourselves trying to get a baby to stop crying and go to sleep. When our baby cries, alarms go off. Our vigilant new-mother brain believes there is something wrong with our baby and—especially when we can't get the crying to stop—wrong with us. This is not entirely rational.

And you know what else isn't exactly rational? The immense love we feel for a small being who cries long and often and sleeps only in spurts, bringing us to our knees and disabling that part of our brain that can think clearly and creatively.

Even in the case of the easiest of babies, there are moments when you've tried everything and your baby is STILL crying, and you realize there is nothing more you can do. And for many mothers, that time comes around quite often, especially in the third month of babyhood.

You Can't Take the Credit for a Happy Baby ...

Some babies cry more and sleep less than others. And there are some who cry less and sleep more. We're here to tell you that neither scenario has much to do with what sort of mother you are. We'd love to say that you can take credit for a cheerful baby, but you can't. Gratitude and humility are the only honest paths for the mothers of good sleepers. You might think it's the swaddling or that special way of rocking him, but most likely it's just his temperament. It's just who he is. And it will change! Fussy babies become self-soothing toddlers. And, by the same token, easygoing babies become irritable preschoolers. It's just the way of human development. Everything—the good and the bad—*is temporary*. It's essential to take on this reality, to internalize it, and to make it your own. It's essential to know that the baby in your arms is every bit as dynamic and evolving as you are, and that the two of you are in motion, that this moment is only a moment. This moment is temporary. There's another one—an entirely different one—on the horizon.

We live in a culture that holds mothers responsible for a baby's behavior and habits, when in truth, a baby affects a mother just as profoundly as a mother influences her baby, if not more so. A baby with an easy temperament is *very* rewarding to care for. They settle easily and quickly and are more predictable with eating, sleeping, and pooping. They can leave a mother feeling pretty good, feeling capable. They can make a new mother think, *I've got this.* And the more often a mother feels this way, the more confident she becomes. It's a positive feedback loop. And it's a feedback loop that a mother's brain is wired for. Postpartum brain changes have made you more vigilant and sensitive to your baby's cries, more intent in your desire to care for her. And those brain changes also make you feel *deeply* rewarded by being able to quiet and soothe your infant. Over time, this positive feedback leads to a sense of accomplishment, of a growing mastery.

… And You Can't Take the Blame for a Fussy One

Mothers of babies who are harder (or impossible) to soothe don't get that same brain feedback, that sense of deep accomplishment, even if they are working just as hard (or harder!) than mothers whose babies are easily calmed. Instead, they feel unraveled, exhausted, and lonely. They feel like failures.

If your baby is one of the many babies who cry a lot, you are not a failure.

Let's say it again: *you are not a failure.*

If you can let this sink in, it can begin to set you free. Free from embarrassment, guilt, and isolation. It can set you free you from rushing around ceaselessly searching for reasons why your baby cries more than other babies. Searching for what you are doing wrong.

We know how hard it can be to accept the fact that you aren't doing anything wrong. It's so hard to let ourselves off the hook and to admit that we might not be able to do much about the crying. And then there's that new-mother brain to contend with, the one that is built to crave the reward feelings we get when we quiet a baby. If your baby isn't so responsive to your marvelously attentive, creative, and loving care, then your brain isn't doing much in the confidence-building department. When you think about it, it seems terribly unfair.

And then, as if all that isn't enough, there's grief, too. The grief over what your baby's infancy, that once-in-a-lifetime experience, maybe just *isn't* going to be.

Erin's first baby was a real crier. We mean a *real* crier. Hours and hours of crying. She and her wife tried everything: car naps, hours of bouncing her on a yoga ball, putting her car seat on top of the dryer, wearing her in a sling, in a Bjorn, in an Ergo. Erin danced; her wife did deep knee bends. Nothing really worked. All the hours of crying were hard. But the hardest part was that Erin had to let go of the idea she had about what motherhood would be for her. She wanted—all she wanted—was to push her baby in a stroller into a coffee shop, order a coffee, and sit and drink the coffee while her baby slept in the stroller.

She didn't need to do it every day, or even that often. She just wanted to do it once. But her baby was not a sit-in-the-stroller kind of a baby. For months she mourned that cup of coffee. And, mourning that cup of coffee, she was really mourning the ideas she had about what kind of mother she would be.

One of the many complicated things about early motherhood—these months when you are existing in the world as a very different person (and also very much the same person) as you were before your baby was born—is that the sort of mother that you are is so relative to the sort of baby you have. Or, to be more accurate, the sort of mother that you *feel* that you are, that you *perceive* yourself to be.

If you have a baby who's not so easy to soothe, you're up against a lot right now: your own ideas about what motherhood would be like, along with a society that's telling you it's time to get things "back to normal"—whatever that means. And, as if that's not enough, you have a nervous system on high alert (mostly unnecessarily) and a brain that really, really wants you to get that baby to stop crying.

Erin has a habit (and she might not be alone in this) of driving far out of her way to avoid traffic. She doesn't necessarily get to where she's going any faster—and she definitely uses more gas—but it feels better than sitting in traffic. She likes to keep moving. This is often how new mothers approach time with a fussy baby. We cajole, shush, dance, nurse, and bounce, when maybe, just maybe, the baby is going to quiet and fall asleep on her own time, no matter what we do. A fussy baby who is sated and dry really might just need your company. Can you offer her that? And can you free up some of your heroic caretaking/ troubleshooting/consoling energy so that you can offer it to yourself?

Can you sit in the psychic traffic with your crying baby so there's some gas left in the tank for you? Can you remember that *it's temporary?*

Did You Know ...

Infant crying from two weeks to twelve weeks is so common that it has been dubbed the "Period of PURPLE Crying," PURPLE being an acronym for crying that *Peaks* around two months and comes on *Unexpectedly.* Your baby is *Resistant* to soothing and looks to be in *Pain,* even though she likely is not. The crying *Lasts* for a long time, mostly in the *Evening.* All this might sound familiar to you.

There are 1.5 million search results when you Google "persistent infant crying," but very few are about the impact crying has on mothers. Christy Clancy, in her story "Colicky Residue," from the anthology *So Glad They Told Me: Women Get Real about Motherhood,* describes her experience of living through colic: "Colic is three months of root canals, jack hammers, metal music, nails on chalkboard, forks scraping against teeth, tea kettle whistles, horns honking, alarms blaring, raging seas. Colic is extreme parenting when you're least ready for it—you're sleep deprived, sagging, leaking, bleeding, engorged, insecure. It was an experience that penetrated every border of patience and sanity that I thought I could maintain."

Our baby's cries are designed to get us to respond, and respond we do! Because we don't often know why our babies are crying, we exhaust ourselves trying everything to soothe and quiet them. And when we can't find a way to soothe them, we're sure there is something wrong— with them, or us. And if we are one of the one in five mothers with a baby who cries for hours a day, every day, for weeks on end, we are sure the world will judge us as a bad mother. Or dole out unsolicited advice.

One of the few interview studies of mothers with so-called colicky babies showed that pediatricians often told them it wouldn't last forever and showed them the door, yet everyone on the street and in restaurants and grocery stores had admonitions and advice. These mothers ended up hiding from all this advice and judgment, further exacerbating the situation by making them isolated and lonely. All they wanted was support and empathy, not advice. They felt they had lost something precious: the quiet baby they had for the first week after birth, the still-sleepy baby who slept and fed, then slept again. And equally as precious, they felt they'd lost the mother they'd thought they'd be.

Crying Baby Tonglen

When a break from a crying baby just isn't possible, *crying baby tonglen* is a practice that works on the spot to help you feel better, something that can sidestep the brain's desire for that feeling of reward and accomplishment, something that helps your nervous system to rest a little, to move your consciousness outside its ardent yet arbitrary ideas of failure and success and into the present moment.

Crying baby *tonglen* is adapted from the ancient Tibetan practice of *tonglen,* which means "receiving and sending." Because it's a breathing practice, it can help you get out of your rushing mind and into your body. Because your instinct is to flee or get the crying to stop, at first it might feel strange to just be with the exhaustion and crying.

As you inhale slowly, allow the situation to be what it is. Acknowledge it all: the crying, the exhaustion, the disappointment, and the annoyance. Breathe it all in. Soften the front of your body. As you exhale, send compassion to you and your baby. Imagine, as if from a small distance, the two of you doing the best you can under the circumstances, knowing that *it's temporary.*

Repeat this two more times.

As you repeat the practice, visualize all the other mothers in the world who are caring for a crying baby and send them some compassion too. You are not alone.

One Minute Yoga 3

GRACE 3

♦ *Gather* yourself in child's pose (shown below) or sitting or lying down. Bring your awareness inward to the sensation of ground, feel yourself connecting to the steadiness of it.

- *Rest* by rolling your shoulders in circles three times in each direction, shake out arms and hands, then just let them sink down while you breathe slower and deeper.

- *Ask* "How am I right now?"

- *Compassion* can take many forms. This month, ask for what you need. Protect yourself from unnecessary obligations.

- *Engage* in your day, knowing that this is temporary. Begin again.

Breathing 3

Continue with *tonglen.*

Use the three-part breath while breathing in any discomfort or anxiety, breathing out ease and peace. Visualize yourself in a large circle of other mothers faced with challenges, all wishing you and each other ease, peace, and happiness.

Asana 3

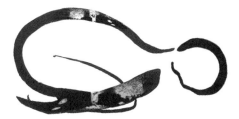

If you are a mother whose baby is crying most of the time, and you can't find quiet moments, simply practice crying baby *tonglen* in child's pose and slow down your movements as you care for your baby. Next month, when things are easier, you can continue with the asana practices. We are sending you a big hug.

If you do have a few minutes while your baby is asleep or happy, cat/cow warm up gives you a chance to reconnect with your body, breath, and movement—with pleasure and a sense of playfulness.

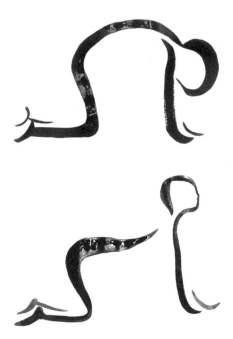

- ♦ Start in child's pose.

- ♦ Kneel and sit back on your heels, then place hands on the floor in front of you and slowly slide them forward until your forehead is on the mat or blanket. You can keep your hands under your forehead or straighten your arms down by your sides. Feel your belly expanding and emptying against your thighs as you breathe.

- ♦ Bring yourself up onto hands and knees: hands under shoulders, knees under hips for cat/cow.

- ♦ Inhale and soften your belly as you lift the tailbone and crown of your head, gently looking upward.

- Allow your lower back to gently arch downward as your chest opens.

- On a nice long exhale, tuck the tailbone under, round your spine toward the ceiling and engage your belly button toward the spine, and lower your head.

- After a few rounds, slow the movements down a lot. Slow is nourishing, slow feels good.

- Move your hips and shoulders very slowly in any way that feels good right now. Play around with your breath, stretch, yawn, and sigh.

- Come back into child's pose and notice how you feel. Before returning to engage with your life, take a moment to repeat this mantra: "It's temporary."

This practice is a way to begin experimenting with slowing down. When you start thinking about your baby's crying as something that isn't your fault, something you can't always fix, you can work on slowing down. And if you can't slow your mind down right away, try consciously slowing down your body, noticing what it feels like to rush. Ask yourself: *What am I rushing toward?* Try moving more slowly. Change a diaper half as fast; wash your face slowly. Walk—don't run— back into the house when you forget your keys. And then notice how it makes you feel.

Maybe you've heard of the slow food movement, so how about slow motherhood?

Mantra 3: It's temporary.

Part Two

MotherSelf
The Fifth Trimester

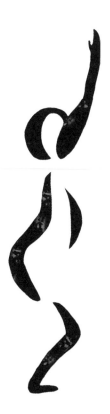

Ambivalent means more than just mixed feelings. It means a love for two things, a love divided. It means a love that moves in two directions, that acts on us in different ways, that brings us different kinds of joy.

Chapter 4

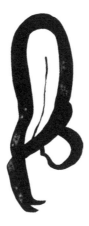

Finding Your Feet

It was Carly who suggested the three of them get together. "Just like old times!" she'd said in her group text.

Funny to think that just four months ago was old times, but considering how much had changed, it *did* feel like old times. Four months ago they were The Bumps, three coworkers who'd found out they were pregnant at the same time. Amber was the sickest of all in her first trimester and couldn't even walk into the office break room without throwing up. So, in solidarity, they all ate their lunches outside on a picnic table behind the building. It was true solidarity, considering it was December. They felt so lucky to have each other. They spent their lunches talking about everything (how often they peed, what smelled good, what smelled terrible) and asking each other all the questions: Are you going to circumcise if it's a boy? Do you think you'll co-sleep? Or nurse?

But then, after the babies were born, after the congratulatory "OMG! She's beautiful!" texts, they lost touch.

Work was suddenly so distant for all of them. They worked at a women's health nonprofit, where the benefits were good (in part because the pay was not), including six full months of maternity leave. They'd been busy with visits from parents and in-laws, baby-and-me exercise classes, and so on. They just hadn't seen each other.

But then came Carly's text: "Hey! We need to give this group a new name! Suggestions?"

Noelle was the first to text back. "How about The Lumps?"

That got everyone going, with lots of crying-laughing emojis and "I've missed you all!" and "OMG, do we need to talk!"

And so they made a date. The weather was still warm, and they decided that, in honor of their first-trimester alfresco lunches, they'd meet outside, at a park near their old office.

Carly arrived first, lay down a blanket, and plopped her baby, a round and cheerful girl, down on it.

Then Amber came, a baby boy strapped to her chest in a wrap. She threw her arms about Carly, and the baby promptly started to cry. "And here we go," Amber said. "This kid has two speeds: crying and about to start crying."

"You're heeeerrrre!"

Carly and Amber turned to see Noelle running toward them—actually running—with a jogging stroller.

Carly and Amber waved, and Carly leaned over to Amber. "I thought you weren't supposed to put a baby in one of those yet," she whispered. "Isn't it six months?"

"I have no idea," Amber whispered back. "I can't even get this boy to sit in a car seat without shrieking. At the rate I'm going, I'll be taking him to kindergarten in this thing." Amber was trying to sound laid back, but the truth was she was pretty close to losing her mind about how much her baby cried and how sad she was that she couldn't just put him in a jogging stroller and take off for a run. Or even a walk. Anything, as long as the baby was quiet.

"This is such a treat!" Noelle said, then took a long swig from her water bottle.

Oh, water! thought Carly. *Damn, I knew I'd forgotten something.* Why was it still so impossible to get out of the house with everything she needed?

Wow, Noelle looks really good, thought Amber. *You've really got to start exercising,* she told herself. Last month she'd downloaded a whole slew of "Mommy and Me" workouts and told herself she'd do one every morning, but she hadn't even done one. The most exercise she got was from bouncing the baby up and down on a yoga ball to get him to go to sleep.

"Sit, sit!" Carly said. "Let's see these babies!" They all sat down on the blanket. "Wow," Carly said, watching as Amber put her baby down on his stomach only for him to roll right over onto his back, then onto his stomach again. "That's amazing." Just this morning Carly had cried to her mom on the phone because her baby wasn't rolling over yet. Now she was sure there was something really, really wrong with her.

"I think she's hungry," said Carly, scooping up her baby, afraid that one of the moms would comment on her inability to roll over. She lifted her shirt, and the baby started to nurse. The sight of Carly nursing made Noelle panic. After mastitis in both breasts and a week of thrush, she'd stopped nursing, and she felt terrible about it. And she also felt terrible, honestly, about how completely relieved she'd been. But she didn't want her friends to know.

"So, Bumps," Amber said, trying to sound cheerful, "how's it going?"

"Great!" Noelle and Carly lied, in unison.

~ ~ ~

> *Don't surrender all your joy for an idea*
> *you used to have about yourself that isn't*
> *true anymore.*
>
> —CHERYL STRAYED

~ ~ ~

The fourth trimester has come to a close. Your baby is still small, and your experience of motherhood is still new, but you are both different beings than you were in those early days after birth. You've figured out a few things. Your baby is more alert, more human.

This is a good time to talk about this idea of "getting your life back." It's a fraught concept and, we think, a misleading one. So much of the talk of life with a baby after the first three months is about what you can get *back*. What you can return to or regain. But birth and early motherhood alter us in such profound ways that we think it's helpful to focus less on *returning* and more on *moving forward*. This isn't to say that we don't understand (or remember oh so well) the idea of wanting to get back our bodies, our minds, our good night's sleep. We do! It's just that birth and babies change *everything*, and in the face of that fact, we think it can be more satisfying, self-affirming, and—honestly—more fun to think about moving your body, mind, relationships, sleep patterns, and everything else forward. Forward into a new world, a new life, and new ideas about yourself and what you are capable of, what you need, and what really matters to you.

Of course, it can be just as important to connect with people and experiences from life before baby that are grounding. A silly (but important) example: When Erin's first baby was three months old, she threw out her sensible black diaper bag and replaced it with an impractical hot-pink leather handbag because it made her feel like herself again. The straps didn't fit over her shoulder, the bag had no good pockets, and she could never find anything in it, but that bag brought her back to herself. That bag made her happy.

So perhaps what we're trying to say here is that this transition is a time of moving forward *as well as* bringing your most beloved parts of yourself from before birth forward with you, instead of trying to get your new reality to move "back" to before.

When *You* Feel Ready

In keeping with this idea of moving forward into the fifth trimester, our yoga practice this month will be a transition from floor to standing. Transitions bring feelings of uncertainty, loss, and excitement. They also lead to transformation.

In yoga, a teacher often moves the class into a new posture by saying, "And when you feel ready ..." *When you feel ready* is an important cue in yoga and in life as a mother. The transitions of the fifth trimester—transitions to work, to more time away from your baby, to new sleeping arrangements—all start when you feel ready, not because you have now reached a particular postpartum month. You might want to stay where you are for a while longer; you might even need to take a step back. And if you do, know that it's perfectly fine to scale back and rest if you've taken on more than you have energy for. In a yoga class, you can always move out of a straining pose right into child's pose, and you can stay there as long as you need to. The same goes for life with a baby. You can adapt schedules, routines, or anything that's putting too much of a strain on you right now. You can step back from trying to nurse your baby while taking a work call or squeezing a trip to the grocery store between two naps. If your transition is too much right now, *if you need more time,* remember that child's pose, however you might define it, is always waiting.

Of course, it's also possible that you were ready and eager to get back to work, activity, socializing, travel, and the adult world in general long before this time. Regardless of where you're at, we think it's fairly likely you feel some ambivalence. Which is why we think this is a good time to slow down, take a closer look at these transitions, and think about how you might want to move through them. Like transitions in our yoga practice, transitions in life go better if we move slowly, break it down, and tune in to the way we feel from the inside out.

You are moving out of what Alison likes to call the "mother-baby couple bubble" phase. Your attention is naturally beginning to turn outward as you take on more responsibilities and face new decisions about work, friends, and activities.

Step Away from the Instagram

It's normal at this pivotal point to be asking, *Who am I now?* And in trying to answer that question, it's tempting to create unrealistic expectations for you and your baby. These expectations are often fueled by comparisons with other mothers, both in person and on social media. When we compare our private self to someone else's public self, we get a distorted comparison. Be especially wary of comparing yourself to anyone who is trying to manage the impression they are making. And, quite honestly, that's every mother—celebrity moms, Instagram moms, the moms in your baby group, your sister-in-law who had a baby a few weeks before you did. New mothers are uncertain and vulnerable, and the world is filled with judgment toward them. So of course new moms are trying to manage the impression they're making, trying to present a cohesive, capable self and a happy, content baby.

Which is what makes these comparisons especially harmful. As a friend of Erin's once said, "The comparison game is the only game we play to lose." And it's true—we often seek images or ideas of motherhood that end up making us feel badly about ourselves.

A more gentle, nurturing way to compare your private mother self to another private self is to read literature about motherhood, written by mothers, like *Operating Instructions* by Anne Lamott and *Things I Don't Want to Know* by Deborah Levy. Such books can give us a sense of connection and empathy with these authors, and they can also illuminate parts of our experience that perhaps we weren't aware of.

Another way to feel connection is to be brave enough to share your own imperfections and vulnerability, to take a break from managing the impression you're putting forward. In one of Alison's workshops, a mother answered the question "What brought you here?" with a story of a recent morning at her home. She was in the kitchen, with her toddler on her hip, when her phone rang. She went to grab the phone, and her toddler's foot knocked a dozen eggs onto the floor. She yelled something really satisfying yet crude, and the dog came rushing in the open door and slid into home base through the eggs. Starting to cry and laugh, she peed in her pants. This, she said, was the reason she had come to the workshop. She thought she could use some yoga.

One by one, through tears and laughter, every mother told the real story of her life, not the Instagram version, not the good impression. Sitting in that circle, with the truth shared and exposed to light, there was a collective sigh of relief. This was the first time some of these mothers had felt safe sharing the stories of their inner lives. Many mother-and-baby groups had felt more like a competition to these women, leaving them more isolated than ever. That one brave mother gave the rest of the group permission to relax and open up. And in that moment, all of the mothers felt connected and realized that they weren't alone and weren't the only ones feeling isolated, insecure, and overwhelmed.

Every Mother Needs a Friend Like Alison (Says Erin)

Our third suggestion is perhaps our favorite: befriend an older mother, someone whose children are grown or at least much older than yours. We know it isn't easy to find a friend outside your demographic, but book groups, yoga classes, and spiritual communities can all be places to start. Erin and Alison's friendship (which began when Alison joined a Peace and Justice study group with Erin's then girlfriend, now wife) was a source of comfort, wisdom, and much hilarity for Erin in her early days of motherhood, and it continues to be that fifteen years later. When Alison came over to meet Erin's baby for the first time, the baby was sleeping, and Erin couldn't stop looking at the clock. "She needs to eat in five minutes," Erin said. "I need to wake her up." Alison peered over the side of the bassinette at the sleeping baby. "She looks pretty happy right now," she said. "How about you just eat some of that cake I brought, and we wait for her to wake up?"

Every mother needs a friend like Alison, someone who can tell you not to wake your sleeping baby and also regale you with stories about the time she and her husband took their three-month-old to an island in Maine, and she rinsed her cloth diapers by hand and then boiled them. (True story! Alison boiled cloth diapers! Then hung them on a clothesline that she'd strung herself between two trees!) And together you can laugh; you can laugh so hard about boiling diapers in pursuit of perfect motherhood. Because if a friend your own age told you that same story, well, you might have a lot of feelings about her and her diapers, and she might have a lot of feelings about her and her diapers: jealousy, inadequacy, judgment, annoyance, and defensiveness, just to name a few. But when a woman a generation (or two) beyond tells a story of too-earnest maternal striving, you can laugh. And laughter is one of the most powerful forces we have to create the momentum we need to move forward into a meaningful and enjoyable life with a baby.

More specifically, *your* life with *your* baby. In your time.

Motherhood Is a Relationship

When we compare ourselves to others, we are looking away from ourselves and our babies. One of the keys to that sense of meaning and enjoyment we want to be moving toward in the fifth trimester is to think differently about what, exactly, motherhood is, and to claim your own motherhood experience. At this particular transition time, it's helpful to move away from the idea of motherhood as an identity toward the idea of motherhood as a relationship. A rich, unique relationship between you and your baby, one that will continue to evolve as your child grows. And one that will move at your own pace, in your own time.

In earlier chapters, you started to become familiar with ways to calm and soothe your nervous system with your breath and self-compassion. Now we can go one step beyond those calming practices to a practice of gentle awareness and curiosity about yourself and your baby.

Start by gently observing your baby as she is now. It's always easier to observe someone other than yourself at first. How much stimulation does your baby like? Does she like being outdoors or around lots of people, or does she prefer the quiet of home? Does she need routines, or is she adaptable to change? Does she feed quickly and efficiently or does she like to take her time, interacting with you? How does she do with other caregivers?

Now turn your attention to yourself, using the same nonjudgmental approach. Are you craving company, or does company wear you out? Are you aching to take on a project, or would a bath feel better? Are there moments when you feel content, capable, and expansive, and others when you feel confused, overwhelmed, and contracted? The more you can observe the ways in which you are responding to the demands of your relationship with your baby, the easier it will be to sort out what feels good and important, and what is causing you anxiety or creating a sense of dissonance. You can notice what gets you up and moving and what settles and grounds you. The more you listen to these messages within, the less distracted you will be by unrealistic expectations and comparisons.

Mothers Are Our Heroes, but They Are Not Superheroes

One Halloween, many years ago, a sweet little boy we knew dressed up as Superman. He'd been looking forward to the day for months, and his mother had made him a wonderful costume. On Halloween night he put it on, looked in the mirror, and was crestfallen. "What's wrong?" his mother asked. "I thought I was going to be Superman," he said, tears in his eyes, "but I'm just a jerk in a cape."

No matter how old we are, sometimes it can feel like there's an unbridgeable gap between who we are and who we think we should be. This sense that we aren't enough leaves us anxious and disappointed. Often the expectations we have for ourselves and our babies far exceed what is realistic. This can be a good time to ask: What sort of superhero abilities do I expect of myself? To always meet my baby's needs? To be at ease in the face of motherhood's twin states of profound responsibility and deadening monotony? To be entirely confident in my baby's attachment to me, never worried or anxious about the hours she spends in the care of others? And then, when you fail to perform at superhero levels, do you feel like a jerk in a cape? You're not! You're a mother trying to reconcile deeply held expectations with an unexpected new reality. This is one of the reasons so many new mothers feel anxious. When who you are and what you think you should be are pretty much the same thing, there's peace. There's contentment. But in the early months of motherhood, expectation and reality can exist on opposite sides of a canyon. The first step to narrowing that divide comes with shifting your gaze away from others and toward yourself and your baby. It comes with a close and affectionate look at your feelings.

Feelings Are Great Messengers

We can tune into sensations in the body that are associated with feelings. We can notice the stories we tell ourselves and the feelings they evoke. You may notice a whole new menu of feelings since becoming a mother. Feelings are pretty fleeting, but often without even knowing it, we are working overtime to avoid or resist certain feelings, especially boredom, anger, and anxiety. What would happen if you just allowed for anxiety from time to time? Or we might be chasing other feelings, like pleasure or connection. The more aware we are of the feelings that motivate us, the more freedom we have to choose our responses to those feelings. Read over the list of feelings below and notice what your response is to each one.

acceptance	confidence	curiosity
anger	connection	disappointment
anxiety	contentment	embarrassment
boredom	courage	empathy

enthusiasm	grief	love
fear	guilt	regret
frustration	jealousy	resilience
generosity	joy	sorrow
gratitude	loneliness	vulnerability

Now, in real, moment-to-moment life, especially life with a baby, we experience many emotions at once, and they are often contradictory. As you most likely already know, it's possible to feel both terribly bored and completely enamored with your baby. In chapter 5, we'll talk about the intense ambivalence inherent in all mother-baby relationships and how to keep moving forward in the face of conflicting and confusing emotions. But first, it's important to practice simply identifying those oft-conflicting feelings, a practice that will gently but firmly require you to shift your attention away from the compelling distraction of other mothers, both on social media and in real life, and focus on yourself and your baby. Your attentive, noticing mind can't be in two places at once. Let us clarify that: your noticing mind *can try* to be in an endless number of places at once, but it can only succeed at being in one place at a time. And right now that place needs to be your own heart.

Because your motherhood is about you. You and *your* baby. *In your own time.*

Did You Know ...

Accepting ambivalence can set you free. And it can free up energy that would otherwise go into denying feelings. We live in a world where ambivalence about motherhood is prohibited. Mother's voices of regret are silenced. It is perfectly normal to feel ambivalent about everything from the pain of childbirth to breastfeeding to the constant and unrelenting demands of baby care. The less support we have, the more ambivalence we are likely to feel. When we don't have adequate help, we have fewer resources to go around, and competition for our time and energy is more intense. Imagine how your feelings about breastfeeding would change if you had another person to do all the cooking and housework for you? Most of us, sadly, don't have that kind of help, so we are usually exhausted and conflicted while loving our baby more than we could have imagined.

If we can accept ambivalent feelings as a normal part of motherhood, not something to be overcome, hidden, or denied, we can free ourselves. We free ourselves to simply feel what we feel. And then let it pass. It is normal. So you might want to come to your feet and move out into the world, and at the same time, you might want to just lie on the bed and stare at the miracle that is your baby. The more you allow yourself to feel both of these emotions compassionately, without fighting either, the sooner an impulse in one direction or the other will surface. *In your own time.*

One Minute Yoga 4

GRACE 4

In child's pose:

- ♦ *Gather* your attention and energy inward in child's pose, by feeling your shins and hands on the floor and your belly on your thighs.

- ♦ *Rest and relax* your shoulders, jaw, and belly as you breathe three slow, deep breaths.

- ♦ *Ask* "How do I feel right now?" "Where do I feel it in my body?" "What emotions am I feeling now?" "What emotions am I avoiding, wishing for?"

- ♦ *Compassion* is the ability to listen to the answers with curiosity, without judgment, the way you would listen to a dear friend.

- ♦ *Engage* with your life with more ease, curiosity, and acceptance. Begin again.

Breathing 4

In child's pose or while moving, focus your attention on your inhale, without speeding it up or deepening it unless you want to. Feel fresh new oxygen filling your lungs. Allow the exhale to just happen. Repeat for three breaths.

Asana 4

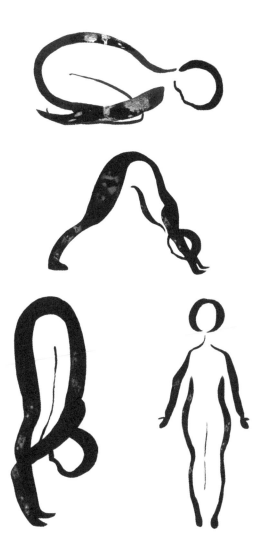

- Come into child's pose.

- Take three slow, deep breaths, focusing more on the inhale, and allowing the exhale to just happen.

- If you're feeling ready to come to standing, then, on the next inhale, lift your hips to the sky into downward-facing dog. Bend your knees and lengthen your spine. Take three long, slow breaths in downward-facing dog. Let your heels drop a little toward the mat or peddle your feet gently.

- Walk your feet slowly toward your hands, knees bent, foreword fold, sway side to side for one or two breaths.

- On the next inhale, bring your hands to your thighs, flatten your back, engage your core and hinge from your waist like a clamshell, coming up to standing. Exhale. Take a long, deep breath and let your shoulders soften down. Feel your body standing up. Notice whatever you are feeling from your feet to your crown.

Mantra 4: In my own time.

Chapter 5

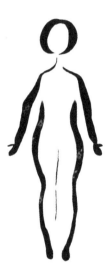

Mountain Pose

When Adia was pregnant, she read a magazine profile about a writer who worked with her infant in a stroller next to her desk. When the baby started to stir, the writer would just jiggle the stroller with one hand and type with the other. "I've never been more productive," the writer said, "because now I don't have any time to procrastinate. When the baby is quiet, I'm working. No excuses."

That will be me, thought Adia. When my baby is quiet, I'll be working. No excuses. Of course, Adia had never really wanted an excuse to not work. She loved her job, and she had no intention of giving it up when the baby was born. She also loved the idea of being with her baby. And she knew she could do both. If that writer could do it, so could she.

"So you're a graphic designer," Adia's midwife said during one of her second trimester visits.

"Yes," Adia replied, "and I own my own company, which means I'll be able to work from home, with the baby."

"Oh, I wouldn't count on that," the midwife said, with a kind smile that struck Adia as a little smug. "There's not much time for work with a new baby."

"Well, I guess I'll see," Adia said, taking the midwife's doubt as a challenge. "I'll just see how it goes."

~ ~ ~

In the first three months of her baby's life, Adia thought of that midwife every time she sat down to work. *You were so wrong,* she thought as the baby slept next to her desk in a bassinet. In fact, Adia began working a few hours every day when her baby was only a month old. She was deeply proud of what she'd managed to do—to maintain her clients, do good work for them, and take care of her baby.

Until the day she couldn't.

~ ~ ~

"Sleepy, sleepy, little bunny," Adia sang as she bounced on a yoga ball, the baby strapped to her chest. She kept looking at the time on her phone. 10:05 a.m. 10:17. 10:31. The baby's naptime came and went, and still the baby showed no sign of going to sleep. She chortled, blew spit bubbles, grabbed onto Adia's hair and pulled, hard. All the while, Adia was trying to work. Trying and failing. "Time for sleep! All the sweet little baby bunnies are asleep!" Adia sang in a high-pitched, not-at-all-calming voice as she tried to reach around the baby and type a long-overdue email to a client. She was having trouble remembering what she wanted to say because she was so queasy from all the bouncing.

Finally, Adia gave up. She took the baby out of the sling, put her in the stroller, and headed out the door, hoping that a walk around the block might do the trick. As she walked, she called her boyfriend. "Can you come home for a few hours so I can finish this project?" she asked. "It's due at five."

"Sorry, hon, I can't. I'm short two staff today."

"Well, I'm short on staff today too," Adia said curtly.

"You know," her boyfriend said. "I think it's probably time."

"For what?" Adia asked, feeling defensive.

"For some childcare," her boyfriend said. "We need to do our jobs, and this bring-your-work-to-baby thing isn't working anymore."

"But we said six months!" Adia said.

"Or whenever we needed it," her boyfriend reminded her. "And I think we need it."

"I can't leave her. What if I hired a babysitter to come here and be with her while I work?"

"Where would you work?"

"I could convert the laundry closet into an office," she suggested.

"Look, hon, maybe we should just interview some people."

"But I don't want to be away from her!" Adia cried.

"Well, then maybe we should think about you cutting back."

"I don't want to cut back! And we can't afford to," Adia cried.

"I don't know what to say," Adia's boyfriend said, "but I think something's gotta give."

~~~

When she is with them she is not herself; when she is without them she is not herself; and so it is as difficult to leave your children as it is to stay with them.
—RACHEL CUSK, *A LIFE'S WORK*

~~~

We often hear women say that they are feeling ambivalent about returning to work after having a baby. *Ambivalent* is a word we often associate with mixed feelings, hesitation, or even disinterest.

But *ambivalent* means more than just mixed feelings. It means a love for two things, a love divided. It means a love that moves in directions, that acts on us in different ways, that brings us different kinds of joy.

As you find your feet and begin to stand tall in mountain pose, it's a good time to expand your ideas about ambivalence. It's love pulling you in two different directions, love that makes you wobble, love that moves you in and out of balance. Love is on both sides.

The Not-So-Great News about Childcare in the United States (Which You Probably Already Know)

Remember in the introduction when we cautioned you to stay away from any baby-rearing manual that refers to another country in its title? One of the main reasons for our insistence that these books harm more than they help has to do with childcare in the United States as it compares to childcare around the world. We think the single most constraining, complicating, and downright infuriating aspect of being a mother in the United States today is our country's refusal to create and sustainably fund parental leaves and universally affordable childcare. We believe it is the factor that makes motherhood in France, Germany, Scandinavia, Australia, and a host of other places a fundamentally different experience, one that simply can't be compared with American motherhood. American women's limited access to childcare is yet another example of our country's insistence that women should find a personal solution to what is, essentially, a societal need.

We mention all this only because, as we move forward in our discussion of how to make decisions that work for you and your baby at this stage, we simply want to acknowledge the fact that you are in a tough situation, one that is challenging for emotional and logistical reasons, reasons that you can't control. So as we offer ways to help you navigate those decisions, it's always with the knowledge that mothers who seek childcare for their babies are up against struggles that mindfulness, yoga, and self-compassion might be able to ease, but can't resolve.

Finding and paying for childcare—infant care in particular—is the central struggle of this time with a baby for so many women. A maternity leave, if you even had one, is most likely coming to an end, and there are so many decisions to be made. Nanny or out-of-home care? Childcare center or home-based childcare? Parents or in-laws? Part-time or full?

Love Is on Both Sides, and So Is Desire

Even if you're not on your way back to a paying job right now, you are, most likely, feeling the need (either emotionally or logistically) to spend more time away from your baby. As we think about motherhood as a relationship, this is a good time to remember that in a close relationship we simultaneously want intimacy *and* autonomy. This phase of development as a mother is often marked by your increasing tolerance for small separations from your baby, in sleeping arrangements, time at work for you, and time at childcare for your baby. This increased tolerance, of course, doesn't mean that the transition to work or time away from your baby is easy. Quite the opposite. It might actually create a whole new set of tensions. You may want desperately to focus on your career again, while at the same time find it excruciatingly hard to be apart from your baby for even a few hours at a time. Or you may have decided to stay home with your baby for a while longer, then find yourself resenting the constant demands, isolation, and boredom inherent in life with a baby.

Trying to reconcile these desires is futile and exhausting. Instead, as Bruce Tift suggests in his book *Already Free,* you might need to adopt this mantra: "I give myself permission to feel torn, off and on for the rest of my life without any hope of resolution."

We know it sounds a bit drastic, especially the "without any hope" part, but we think there's something freeing about the absoluteness of Tift's idea. *No way, nope, not a chance.* So you can stop striving and straining and expecting something of yourself that no mother is capable of. And once we start allowing for the simultaneous desire for closeness and separateness with our baby, without trying to fix it, it will be easier to deal with the fact that when you are at work, you long to be home with your baby, and when you are home with your baby, you long to be anywhere else, without him. You will be able to stand securely, like a mountain, in ambivalence. It may be the most liberating stance you can adopt and carry throughout your life as a mother and a partner.

We just can't love our babies the way we do and expect to resolve our desires for closeness and space, to hit a sweet spot. Of course, there will be moments, days, even weeks, where we feel that balance, but then something will change, and we'll feel torn again. Something always changes. What remains constant is our love for our children, our desire to be close to them, and our desire for autonomy. *Love is on both sides.*

Feelings Are Messengers, but Values Are Companions

Let's return to the specific challenge of finding childcare. Many women wanting (or needing, or both wanting and needing) to return to work quickly become angry at the lack of options and support available to them. They may not have enough, or any, paid maternity leave. They may feel anxious that no one can take care of their baby as safely and capably as they can themselves. Or, conversely, they might be excited to get back to work, thrilled with the childcare option they managed to secure, and still be deeply sad to be away from their baby.

Every one of these emotions are messengers, some fleeting, some more enduring, but all, ultimately, are temporary. Additionally, as we mentioned in the last chapter, it isn't unusual to have two competing and compelling feelings simultaneously. We often feel ambivalent about closeness and separateness with our baby. If we want to honor our emotions but not have our choices be dictated by them, how do we make the difficult decisions like childcare arrangements?

We can begin by shifting our attention away from our feelings for a moment, and think instead about our values. Values are different from feelings. Feelings come and go, alter, transform. Values only clarify over time, become more solid and smooth, like a stone in your pocket. If emotions are like clouds in the sky, values are the trees below, trees whose roots will deepen and whose branches will transform with the seasons, but whose trunk will remain, unmoving.

Values aren't goals, in that we never accomplish a value. Instead, values are like a compass—they help us make choices based on the directions we want our life to go. Values are especially helpful in making decisions in challenging or difficult times. Values are highly individual; they are not rooted in what we think we should do but in what we believe to be important in our lives.

Frightened Is a Feeling; Courage Is a Value

So then, what are *your* values now? This is not an easy question, but it is an essential one. Because when you can identify your values, you can acknowledge and respect your emotions, all the while knowing that you need to make big decisions from a different place. The emotions of motherhood are wildly strong, deeply felt, and both enduring and ever changing. They are intoxicating, beautiful, maddening, enlivening, and sometimes debilitating. In other words, they are a rollercoaster. And they can give us so much information about ourselves, provide so many opportunities for self-compassion. What they can't do is help us make decisions.

But values are different. Values do help you make decisions, by orienting you toward the life you want to live. In order to determine your values, you must discover and clarify what matters to you. There are many traditions that can guide you toward an understanding of what you value in life as a new mother. The yogic tradition relies heavily on three values: non-harming, compassion, and kindness. Interestingly, in yoga, there is equal emphasis on non-harming, compassion, and kindness *toward the self* as there is toward others. So if you value

compassion and kindness, it means you value compassion and kindness toward yourself just as much as you value it toward others. We
think this emphasis on mutuality is essential. Anything that you value
for your baby, you must value for yourself too. Any decision you make
needs to work for both of you. If co-sleeping allows your baby to sleep
peacefully but leaves you sleep deprived, undernourished, and tense,
well, according to the mutuality requirement for any decision, co-
sleeping isn't the right decision. Motherhood is a relationship, and in
this relationship your well-being is just as important as your baby's.

Here are some other values new mothers can consider as guide-
posts: courage, reliability, generosity, curiosity, optimism, and flexibility. In thinking about your own values, we encourage you to reflect
on each of these on the list, add any that might be missing for you,
and then pick your top three. Write them on sticky notes, put them
up around your home. Alison likes to write them on index cards and
slip them under her yoga mat; they are then literally the ground she
stands and moves on.

Once you have selected your three most important values, you can
start using them to guide your decisions.

~ ~ ~

Let's go back now and revisit Adia. She had expectations when she was
pregnant about how she would combine motherhood and work. And
then she was lucky for a few months and was recovered enough to be
able to get work done while her baby slept. She naturally didn't want
to have to decide between work and being with her baby. But now she
wants both, and her baby isn't cooperating. Emotionally, Adia is torn
between wanting to be with her baby and doing the work she loves
and having the salary she needs. If she allows her emotions be her only
guide, Aida will continue to feel stuck or will seesaw between contradictory feelings. It's hard to think clearly and make good decisions this
way.

So the first thing Adia will need to do is to take some time to ask
herself, *How am I feeling right now?* off and on throughout the day, and
to ask that question with generosity, kindness, and compassion. She

can take a few minutes to feel the sensations in her body that accompany those emotions. The next thing Adia will need to do is to give herself permission, now that she is a mother, to feel torn, off and on, for the rest of her life, with no hope of resolution. Deep sigh. There is no escaping the ambivalence. There is only the knowledge that there will be some solutions that are better than others, but no perfect one. At least not perfect for more than an hour or a day or maybe, if lucky, a week here and there.

Next, whenever Adia is ready, she could take out her three values cards and ask herself how each of the possible solutions stacks up against her values. Let's say she picks non-harming, compassion, and kindness. She might ask if having her baby in childcare for X number of hours would be non-harming to her and her baby, and would it be a compassionate and kind choice for the two of them. If the answer is yes, she could add that to a list of possible solutions. In this way, Aida will come up with a few solutions to choose from that are aligned with her values and take into account her emotions. She won't find a perfect solution, but she'll probably find one that's good enough for now. No decision with a baby has to be permanent. Most parenting decisions are experiments and should be seen that way. We might need to make modifications in schedules and childcare settings or providers as we tune in to our own development as a mother and that of our baby.

Did You Know …

One reason there are no perfect solutions to the childcare dilemma in the United States is because, as a society, we demand more from workers and offer less family support than any other developed country in the world. It leaves mothers stressed, exhausted, and insecure. And money matters. In the United States, couples spend 25.6 percent of their income on childcare costs, and that number soars to 52.7 percent for single parents, according to the report from the OECD (Organization for Economic Co-operation and Development). The average cost of full-time childcare in the U.S. is $10,000 per year. And the costs vary state to state, depending on subsidies.

There are many choices families make for childcare, from informal care with family members to center-based infant care to pooled nannies. The important thing to consider is the conclusion from the American Academy of Pediatricians which states: "All of a child's early experiences, whether at home, in childcare, or in other preschool settings are educational. The indicators of high quality care have been studied and are available in many formats. When care is consistent, emotionally supportive, and appropriate to the child's age, development, and temperament, there is a positive effect on children and families." In other words, it's not so much the form of childcare but the quality of that care and the fit between the caregiver and infant that matters.

On a lighter note, Harvard University's Kathleen M. McGinn analyzed the results of international surveys and found that not only did the adult daughters of mothers employed outside the home do better in their own careers, but all adult children of employed mothers were just as happy as the adult children of women who had been stay-at-home mothers. And, interestingly, the adult sons of mothers who worked outside the home were more egalitarian as husbands and fathers. A panel of the young adults in one such survey was convened and asked if they had any advice for mothers who worked outside the home, to which every one of them responded, "just chill—we're fine."

So apart from the fact that you would never, for obvious reasons, see a study examining whether children of fathers employed outside the home are as happy as the children of stay-at-home fathers, the message is that the kids will be fine. The authors hope surveys like these will relieve the guilt many women feel as they kiss their child goodbye, so they can go to work. We wish it were so simple—read a survey and relax—but we know it isn't. But maybe, in some small incremental way, it will help mothers feel a little more comfortable with the decisions they make about their work and their child.

One Minute Yoga 5

GRACE 5

- *Gather* your attention and strength in toward your center line by standing with legs a few feet apart, hands on hips. Feel strong, like a mountain, as if you can withstand winds and storms.

- *Rest* with your eyes closed as your shoulders relax down away from your ears.

- *Ask* "What do I value now." Feel that as your base of support.

- *Compassion* this month for the natural ambivalence of motherhood.

- *Engage* with your day with more confidence, courage, and strength. Begin again.

Breathing 5

Inhale to the count of four. Imagine your breath coming up through your roots, up and out your crown.

Exhale to the count of four. Imagine your breath sinking down through your body into the earth.

Asana 5

MOUNTAIN POSE

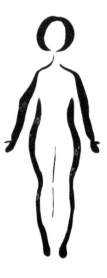

- Stand with feet hip-width apart, hands by your sides. Bring your attention to your feet.

- Notice how your toes touch the ground; now lift them and then lay them back down. How does that feel?

- Come up onto your tiptoes, then bring your heels back down. Does that feel different? If it does, how?

- Imagine you are squeezing a block or ball between your thighs, lengthen your spine, shoulders relaxed, hands by your side, and the crown of your head reaching up toward the sky. Take three slow breaths. You are in mountain pose, strong and stable.

CRESCENT MOON POSE

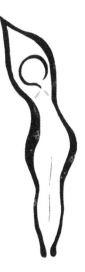

- From mountain pose, with your next inhale, raise your arms up and over your head.

- Relax your shoulders down with an exhale.

- Interlace your fingers over your head and with your hips aligned with the front of your mat, inhale while you lengthen your spine up.

- Exhale, allow your torso and arms to stretch over to the right, feeling the stretch in the left side body.

- Inhale back to center and repeat to the left.

- Come back into mountain pose with your arms by your sides. Notice how you feel.

- Rest in *savasana* or child's pose, if you have time.

Mantra 5: Love is on both sides.

Chapter 6

Awkward Pose

When Eliza agreed to play the cello in her friend's wedding, she could imagine the day perfectly. She would play Bach's cello suites, per her dear friend's request, and her soon-to-be born baby would sleep on a blanket beside her. Or maybe the baby would sleep in the arms of Eliza's wife. Either way, the baby would sleep, and Eliza would play the cello.

But now the day of the wedding has arrived, and the baby isn't sleeping. He's shrieking. Also, Eliza's wife is on a business trip, so

Eliza is alone as she drives through the Blue Ridge Mountains from her home to the once bucolic and now maddeningly remote farm where the wedding will be held. The baby has been screaming since the moment Eliza buckled him into the car seat. This is no surprise to Eliza; the baby hates the car. He screamed the whole way home from the hospital the day after he was born, and he's screamed through every car ride since. Eliza and her wife have done everything they can to avoid getting in the car with him. They've starting having their groceries delivered. Her wife has pushed the baby two miles each way in the stroller to every pediatrician appointment. But Eliza can't push him in a stroller all the way to this wedding. He's just going to have to cry.

Which is just what he does, at first. But soon enough, he's screaming. Eliza knows there's nothing he needs: he's dry and fed. He's sleepy but not overtired. His sunshade is adjusted properly; he's dressed for the weather. She's done all she can. So she keeps driving. She sings to him, sings all the protest songs of her child-hood—"Union Miners Stand Together" and "If I Had a Hammer." She sings some Dolly Parton favorites, "Apple Jack" and "Coat of Many Colors," and then moves onto a rather desperate rendition of "Shenandoah," which under normal conditions has a miracu-lously sedative effect. But not now. Still, Eliza keeps singing, and sweating.

When the crying had been going on for forty-five minutes, and Eliza thinks she can't take another minute, she comes to the terrible realization that home is now farther away than the farm, and there's nothing to do but keep going. She starts to cry. She's so tired. So, so tired. How is it even possible to be this tired? What had she been thinking, embarking on this trip with a six-month-old who hates the car? What in the world could possibly be worth all this crying? But she's promised her friend, and she has to be there. And she's looked forward to it for so long, the chance to play, to make some beautiful music. But she also just wants to go home, to end the baby's—and her—misery. Has she ever been so stuck?

*Life is going to unfold however it does:
pleasant or unpleasant, disappointing or
thrilling, expected or unexpected, all of
the above! What a relief it would be to
know that whatever wave comes along,
we can ride it out with grace.*
—SYLVIA BOORSTEIN

Yes, what a relief it would be to know we could ride life's waves with grace! Surely Eliza would have liked to know that, would have liked to feel that her tense and conflicted ride through the Blue Ridge was something she could handle. Something she *was* handling. *Eliza is so much stronger than she thinks she is.* The trouble is that in early motherhood, we often confuse quiet and calm with mastery and competency. A quiet, content baby means a job well done; a fussing baby means a failure. What if we told you neither is true?

Alison's first baby was, relatively speaking, a breeze, which made her feel like a competent mother. Erin's first baby didn't stop crying until she was three months old, which shook Erin's nascent maternal confidence to its (already wobbling) core. Then we had our second babies (Erin's easier, Alison's more challenging) and realized that it wasn't about us. A baby is not the measure of a mother. Just think about how inconsistent babies are. Happy one minute, shrieking the next; sleeping through the night at three months, multiple night wakings at a year. We can't rely on them to accurately reflect our level of commitment or competence. Sometimes, even when we have made a decision based on awareness of our emotions and our values, things don't go as we hoped they would. Remember there are no "perfect" choices, only ones that are better than others.

Eliza is keeping her promise to play music at her friend's wedding despite how uncomfortable and stressful it will be because she deeply values herself as a musician and as a reliable friend. But even though Eliza was aware of her feelings and made her decision based on her values, she's still going to need resilience to get through the day. Because even when you've done everything you possibly can, things are still going to go badly sometimes. Situations are still going to deteriorate—and quickly. This is when, as the saying goes, the tough get going. This is when we need extra grit and resilience and when we need to really understand just what true resilience is made of. This is when we need to acknowledge, to really absorb, the truth that we are strong enough.

Do You Fight or Fly?

But before we talk about resilience, it might be a good idea to back up a bit and think about how you tend to respond to stress. When life's demands outweigh our psychic resources, most of us go into what psychologists refer to as the stress response: fight, flight, or freeze. Most of us respond to stress in the same way every time we feel overwhelmed. If you have a tendency to fight, you will most likely feel angry and irritated when under stress. If you lean toward flight, you will most likely feel afraid or anxious or restless when you hit a rough patch. And if you freeze, you feel stuck or spacey or numb when stressed. No matter your typical response, most of us don't make great decisions when we are in a state of overwhelm. The more we try to solve the problem, the more intractable it becomes.

Like Eliza, you might sometimes feel trapped. She faced two tangled and opposing needs: the need to soothe her baby and the need to do the exact thing that was making her baby cry. She could just push through, exhausting herself and her baby, or she could pause and ease up her effort. She could take a break and allow her body and nervous system to relax a bit before figuring out what to do next. This isn't easy. Most of us need rescue instructions for our self. This is a good time to return to our mantra from chapter 2 and the words of our favorite Buddhist grandma, Sylvia Boorstein, who had these instructions to herself: "Sweetheart, you are in pain. Relax. Take a breath. Let's pay attention to what is happening. Then we'll figure out what to do." This phrase holds the secret to handling stress *if we can remember it.* This is key. Most of us don't remember it much of the time. But we can learn to remember more often.

It helps if we can become better acquainted with our response to stress, so that we know we are in pain or discomfort or under stress. You could change Sylvia Boorstein's instructions to the simple word *stressed.* You can put a hand on your heart and simply say "stressed" to yourself. Then relax, take a breath, pay attention. And then have a certain faith that with a pause, it will be easier to know what to do next. One of the simplest ways to do this is by practicing with the stress response on the yoga mat, where we can learn about ourselves with less distraction from the outside world.

You might be wondering, with all the real-life opportunities for stress, why would we purposely make ourselves uncomfortable on the mat? We do it so that we can practice finding ease and self-compassion in the awkwardness, with fewer distractions; so that we can keep going even when we don't want to. To help us realize that we are stronger than we think.

Awkward pose is a yoga practice that gives us the opportunity to observe our responses to challenging situations. In awkward pose, we simply sit on an invisible chair. It is, as the name suggests, awkward. It can leave you feeling embarrassed, incompetent, edgy, tense, or unskilled. We practice awkward pose in yoga so we can practice holding ourselves in awkwardness with acceptance and kindness in the safe and private space of our yoga mat. Awkward pose can teach us how we feel and how we resist feelings. Or how we feel bad about even having those feelings.

Another reason we practice being uncomfortable on the mat is because this is a setting where we can safely greet those feelings with curiosity, not the need to fix or change them. When we reach our edge of discomfort, we can back out of the pose and rest, then reenter it when it feels right, having lost nothing. In fact, we've gained some strength by resting. Resting and resuming a pose creates more sustainable strength.

In awkward pose we also practice GRACE, with emphasis on self-compassion and ease. We ground our attention in the body through focus. Focus on how our feet feel on the ground and how our body feels in the pose. Then we breathe, relaxing the jaw and shoulders and hands. We ask ourselves how we feel, body and mind, and greet those feelings with kindness. When we want to, we come out of the pose to rest a bit. Then we reenter it, noticing what's changed.

As life with a baby speeds up, we often can't notice our feelings soon enough to catch the opportunity to pause and reflect. That's normal. It's a skill that gets easier over time, the longer we practice. At first (and for a while) we notice after we've reacted. We say, "Oh, I got stressed there and really flipped out." This isn't a problem. It's actually good news. It means you're growing more aware, learning about yourself.

On the mat, when we notice that we want to come out of the pose, we can practice GRACE. It takes a lot of practice before we can reliably access GRACE off the mat, in the heat of the moment. Alison has been practicing for years, and she still celebrates when she remembers it. Erin's been practicing for far less time than Alison, and she's thrilled when she gets from *G* to *R* before her mind is off and running somewhere else. The last thing we want is for you to have one more thing to feel guilty about not doing, as though GRACE is some sort of Kegels of the mind. If you remember, great. If you realize you didn't remember, that's also great. One thing we know is that it gets easier and comes more quickly off the mat the more we practice on the mat. And even when we are only able to practice GRACE on the mat, we are still giving our nervous system that all-important rest and reset. This alone allows for recovery and thriving.

~ ~ ~

Eliza sees a turnoff ahead, a place to picnic near a river. She slows down, turns onto the gravel. She gets out of the car, takes the baby out of his car seat, and walks down the dirt path to the river. The baby quiets as the heartbreaking aftershocks of his sobs shudder through his little body.

It takes Eliza a little while to stop crying. When she does, she has what she will remember as her first conversation with her son. She holds him up, at eye level. "I think you know this already, but in case you don't, I'm a musician," she says. "It's my job." The baby drools onto her hand in response. She doesn't bother wiping it away. "I'm sorry you hate the car," she continues, "but driving is part of life here on earth, so you're going to have to get used to it." The baby's eyes open wide in an expression that Eliza thinks is either wonder or defiance. She can't tell which.

She kicks off her sandals, and stands in the shallows of the river, in the cool water. She bends down and puts the baby's feet in too, and he pulls up his feet, smiles and hums what she will remember as his first song. Eliza walks to the car, puts the baby in his car seat. He starts to shriek, as loud as ever. Eliza starts the car and pulls back onto the road.

~ ~ ~

Eliza did the most helpful thing she could: she took a break; she stopped. She got out of her thinking mind and into her senses. The sensations of air and water and the sound of her baby's giggles were just what she needed so that she could reenter her life with a bit more ease and to remember that she was strong enough to do what she needed to do.

Did You Know …

"Resilience is about recharging, not enduring," Shawn Achor and Michelle Gielan wrote in the *Harvard Business Review*. Occupationally induced stress (like driving to a job with a screaming baby in the car) without adequate time for recovery doesn't build resilience but rather depletes it. What, then, is recovery? There are two kinds of recovery: internal and external. Internal recovery can take place in the context of caregiving. For mothers, this means finding a way to break the cycle of stress, the way Eliza did, by changing your focus from completion of the goal to rest—however temporary the rest might be.

There are other ways to internally recover. You can follow Sylvia Boorstein's rescue formula by acknowledging that your baby is healthy in all ways but just cries in the car. And you could acknowledge that this crying isn't permanent and that it's not your fault. In other words, you reframe the default mode of over-generalizing ("something is wrong with my baby"), personalizing ("it's my fault my baby doesn't sleep in the car"), or seeing things as permanent ("oh god, she'll be crying on her way to college").

External recovery is a physical break during which you aren't responsible for your baby, for a few minutes or a few hours. Getting on your yoga mat, taking a walk, or playing an instrument are all forms of external recovery. Workaholics never take breaks from work, and it creates an imbalance in their lives. "Mamaholics" never take breaks from motherhood and never take time to recover and thus are always depleted and in stress-response mode.

So, if you want to be resilient, stop. Recharge, don't simply endure. *And know that you are strong enough.*

One Minute Yoga 6

GRACE 6

- *Gather* yourself in the present moment, no matter how difficult, knowing you are resilient. Feel where your body meets the ground.

- *Rest* with a few slow breaths. Inhale through your nose, and exhale through your mouth, slowly. Let unnecessary tension melt away.

- *Ask* "Right now, are my baby and I safe?" Most likely, the answer is yes, so now ask, "Am I trying harder than I need to?"

- *Compassionately* bring your hand to your heart and send yourself some loving kindness for all your efforts in the absence of adequate supports.

- *Engage* with your life knowing that you are resilient. Begin again.

Breathing 6

This month we practice some "locks," or *bandhas,* by inhaling fully and holding the breath while pulling in the perineum and abdominals like a strong Kegel. You can add the chin pressed down on your chest. After the count of four, release and exhale loudly through the mouth, then take a nice long, full inhale and exhale. The benefits of the locks are thought to be derived from compressing and then releasing compression, which increases circulation. Experiment and see how you feel after one or two rounds. Many of us find this practice reenergizing.

Asana 6

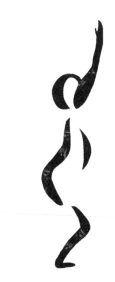

Awkward pose is sometimes called "powerful pose."

- ♦ Take a moment to arrive in standing mountain pose. Bring your attention to your body and feel your feet on the ground, rock back and forth, then sway a little side to side.

- ♦ With hands on hips and with your torso upright and chest lifted, bend your knees and sit back, as if you were about to sit down onto an imaginary chair.

- Bring your arms up by your ears or slightly in front, and breathe.

- Pull your navel in and up.

- Hold the pose for four slow breaths.

- If you need a rest, straighten your legs and stand up for a breath or two and then sink back in.

- Notice how it feels to take a break and then sink back in.

- After four full slow breaths, come out of the pose and shake it out.

- If you have time, come into child's pose or lie down on your back and rest and feel the effects of the pose.

Congratulations. You are learning how to sit in a chair that isn't there and to do it with strength and grace.

Mantra 6: We are strong enough.

Part Three

WomanMother
The Sixth Trimester

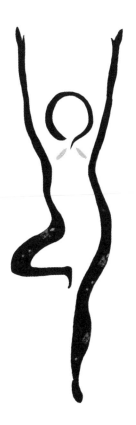

I love my baby more than life itself, but I still love life.

Chapter 7

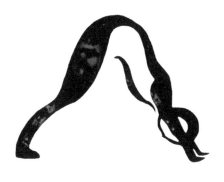

Flow

This year there would be not one but two babies at the Browne family reunion, and as the grandmother of both of those babies, Eileen couldn't have been more excited. Nikki arrived first, with her husband and baby Zadie. When Eileen heard the sound of car wheels on the gravel driveway, she ran out to greet them. "Hello, hello!" she called. "Where's my baby?"

Nikki jumped out of the car. "Shh," she said, bringing her finger to her lips. "Zadie's sleeping." She looked at her watch. "And she needs to stay asleep for twenty more minutes to complete this sleep cycle. Dave will stay with her."

Eileen peered into the backseat car window. "Oh, hon, she'll be fine. Just let me see my granddaughter!"

Nikki steered her mother away from the car. "In twenty minutes," she said. "You can see her in twenty minutes."

"What if she sleeps for thirty?" Eileen asked, meaning it as a joke.

"Oh, Dave knows to wake her," Nikki said, not joking at all.

"He's going to *wake* a sleeping baby?" Eileen asked.

"Don't judge, Mom. It's our system."

Eileen started to say that of course she wasn't judging but then stopped, because, well, maybe she was a little bit, and that wasn't what she wanted to do, not at all. "How are *you?*" she asked instead. "Tell me how you are."

"Terrible," Nikki said. "I thought this was supposed to get easier. I thought I was supposed to feel less exhausted. But now she's seven months old, and I'm as tired as ever, and I'm stressed out."

It was after midnight when the second grandbaby arrived. Nikki and Dave had long since gone to bed, after spending an hour preparing the room where the baby would sleep with room-darkening shades they'd brought from home. Eileen went onto the porch when she heard Maya's car in the driveway. "Hi, Mom," Maya said, getting out of the car. "Sorry we're so late. My god, it takes a long time to get anywhere with a baby."

Eileen hugged Maya. "Where's my grandbaby?" she asked.

Maya gave her a shocked look. "What baby?" she asked, feigning confusion, and then laughed. "He's right here," Maya said, lifting a sleeping and then not sleeping baby out of a car seat. He started to cry.

"Oh, you didn't need to wake him for me," Eileen said. "It's almost one in the morning."

"Is it really? Geez." Maya said, trying to get the baby to take a pacifier he clearly didn't want. "We wanted to get an earlier start, but then I got distracted around the house, and Jared got held up at work, and then I realized we were out of diapers, and—well, you know how it is."

Eileen didn't, not exactly, but she didn't want to say that, not at all. "How are you?" she asked. "Tell me how you are."

"Not great," Maya said. "I thought this was supposed to get easier. But I'm so tired! And you know what else? I'm so stressed out."

~ ~ ~

Yoga is a dance between control and
surrender—between pushing and letting
go—and when to push and when to let go
becomes part of the creative process, part of
an open-ended exploration of your being.
—JOEL KRAMER

Babies Create Chaos

There are two paths parents can take in response to this chaos: we can strive to minimize it through tight controls, schedules, and lots of baby gear, or we can surrender to it, following our baby's cues, going with the proverbial flow. Of course, few of us exist on either extreme of these possibilities, and we can, at different times and different stages, move back and forth between them. It's more helpful to think about your response to baby chaos along a continuum. And wherever you might fall along this continuum, at this time or stage with your baby, schedules are probably on your mind.

If your baby still doesn't sleep much, you are probably putting a lot of effort into ways to engineer some sleep for both of you. Like Nikki, you might have developed some pretty rigid and elaborate strategies that sometimes interfere with other parts of your life. Or maybe you're more like Maya right now, and it feels hard enough to respond to the constantly changing needs of a baby, much less take the time to organize a schedule.

Some of us come to parenting with a tendency toward the rhythmic and regular, a love of structure. Breakfast at seven, a jog every other day, laundry on Saturdays. Even if you weren't so scheduled, chances are you still ate and slept on a fairly regular schedule. But now there's a chaos-maker in your midst, and all that has changed.

For some, structure means comfort and safety; for others, it can feel suffocating and oppressive. The confusing—and paradoxical—thing about structure in life with a baby is that sometimes you need it in order to expand your own sense of freedom. In other words, the more structure in your baby's day, the better your chance for freedom. Erin found that with her second baby; she became an absolute fanatic about her nap. Under no circumstances (okay, under almost no circumstances) would Erin make any plans that would disrupt that afternoon nap. But Erin's rigidity wasn't as much about her daughter's need for sleep as it was Erin's need for writing time and her desire for freedom, for a break from caring for her baby. She needed to create structure in order to experience her own freedom.

But what if your baby's needs don't line up with yours, or what if you can't shape your baby's schedule in a way that works for you? When it comes to living with a baby, it can be really hard to balance your need for structure or your need for freedom from structure with your baby's needs. Can there be a sweet spot of structure for you and your baby when the only constant is change? It is certainly worth investigating.

Not Too Tight, Not Too Loose

The yoga mat is the perfect place to explore our own tendencies and then modify and adjust them until we find the sweet spot between loose and tight, between effort and ease. When you find that moment that feels good, a sweet spot, it feels like an audible sigh—ahhhh. *Not too tight, not too loose.*

Some of us come to our yoga mat with strong, tight calf muscles. We have to slowly stretch and release them to avoid injuring our hamstring and sacrum. On the other hand, if our core is weak, we have to strengthen it to protect our back. That's why we hold in plank position to activate our core muscles before we practice a flow sequence. And then we practice the flow sequence slowly. We take a slow warm up to stretch tight muscles, and we hold postures longer and move between postures slowly and deliberately to build strength. Within the form of yoga there is always room for gentleness. When you discover tightness in downward-facing dog, you can say, "Ah, there it is, a tight calf muscle," and then gently, slowly stretch that tight muscle. Or as you come up to stand from forward fold, you notice a pinch in your lower back and realize your belly muscles weren't engaged. You can try again, gently pulling navel to spine before rising up, protecting your back.

The Goal Is Ease (and Sleep)

Creating schedules or rhythms with a baby isn't that different from the way we explore our bodies on the yoga mat. First we notice how things are now. Then we try something new, we notice again, adjust, notice. Nikki and Maya both arrived exhausted at their mother's house—one sister because she was working overtime to adhere to a schedule, and the other because, lacking a plan, she was constantly reacting to the unpredictable. One a little tight, the other a little loose. Finding the sweet spot means noticing your own and your baby's inherent rhythm and needs and then letting that guide you to create schedules, routines, and rituals *that appeal to you.*

If you are thinking about making changes to the way you schedule your days and nights, it might help to think back to chapter 5 and those central values you identified. Now is a good time to revisit those values, to see if they still provide a solid foundation for decision-making. How would your values inform a new sleep schedule?

You can think of any kind of schedule as a container within which you can practice gentleness and kindness and whatever other values ground your decision-making. The main guiding principle is the question "Am I making things harder for myself, my baby, and my partner?" And if the answer is yes, then the next question is, "How can I make them easier?" The schedule or container you create should help you relax more, not less.

For example, if you decide a bedtime ritual and schedule would be helpful, create one that is as simple or elaborate as you want. Then try it out, and make adjustments. We know one mother who could get through her bedtime ritual in ten minutes with a washcloth, a song, and feeding. Another mother likes to spend at least an hour bathing her baby, massaging her, dressing, reading, singing, feeding, and rocking. She works away from home all day, and bedtime is her way of connecting heart and soul with her baby. Of course, life gets in the way of routines and rituals. There are illnesses, vacations, nights out, growth spurts, developmental shifts. And if, at any time, the need for more sleep becomes the most important goal, ask yourself, "What would be the easiest way to accomplish that?" Then get the sleep, recharge a little, and return to the idea of a schedule or routine again later when you have more resources. Like everything in life with a baby, just as you get used to it, things change. Babies start teething, pulling up to standing in their crib, or having nightmares. So celebrate when you get into a good rhythm, knowing you will find a way to adapt as things shift and change. Always aiming for not too tight and not too loose.

Your Baby Hasn't Read the Manual, So Maybe You Don't Have to Read It Either

There have been debates in the baby-raising literature for years about the relative merits of schedules and routines for babies. These debates tend to be polarized on one end of the spectrum or the other, and they say more about the authors and their time period than they do about the needs of babies and mothers. We recommend that if you use one of the myriad baby manuals on the market today, use it as a tool, not a manifesto. But really, a manual isn't what you need. You have a baby you know and a personal temperament that existed before you became a mother. You have a sense of how regular or spontaneous you naturally are. If you never went to bed at the same time two nights in a row, it's unlikely you will want to now because you had a baby. That said, *your* fluid bedtime might depend on your baby's set bedtime, so that you have the freedom to stay up after she's gone to bed and the freedom to go to bed early because you're tired. Again, it's the paradox of needing a little scheduling for your baby so that you can have a little freedom.

Judith Hanson Lasater, in her book *Living Your Yoga,* tells a story about how hard she, like Erin, tried to create a predictable nap schedule for her children. Just when she thought she had settled on one, her baby's pattern would change. She says she did two things to help herself. She accepted that her baby's nap time wasn't predictable, and then, to create the predictability that she needed for her own sense of well-being, she hired a babysitter for the same few hours every day. That way she had a schedule she could rely on, rather than a schedule that relied on her baby's predictability. She made it easier on her baby and herself.

If you are going to try to make some adaptations, it helps to take a day or two to simply observe yourself, your partner, and your baby, noticing what natural rhythms organically arise. Then you can decide to make adjustments based on observing how exhausted, hungry, and unhappy each of you feels throughout the day. Or, more positively, how rested, nourished, and happy you each feel throughout the day. Then small adjustments can be made, like creating or loosening a bedtime or nap routine. Going back to an illustration from yoga, where not too tight and not too loose is the guiding principle, we can find some helpful tools. We can also talk about these ideas using the terms effort and ease. When we are expending so much effort that we are tense, contracted, and tight, and working so much harder than we need to, we can bring our awareness to our body, and then breathe and relax our shoulders and jaw. This would be the equivalent of Nikki finding herself anxious about her mother wanting to hold her sleeping baby upon arrival. She might notice her own anxiety, breathe, relax, and notice again. And then you do what feels right.

From Structure to Flow: Transitions

In motherhood and in yoga, some structure and predictability provides the freedom to flow more spontaneously. And flowing feels good. One of the most important and less attended to aspects of yoga flow and schedules are the transitions. Those places in-between that bridge one moment or activity to the next. Routines provide a structure for transitions the way strengthening poses provide structure for the transitions in a flow yoga sequence. If we try to rush through transitions without paying attention, it is hard to find flow. Think about the transitions between feeding and walking out the door with your baby. If all you can think about is getting out the door, you might not attend to diapering and dressing your baby, packing up a bag, and so on. You may find, when you've arrived, that you forgot the bag or an extra diaper. In yoga, if you don't pay attention to the transition between forward fold and standing, you can put too much strain on your back, so when you get to mountain pose, you have a tweak in your lower back.

We all tend to be less aware of transitions. It's natural. Focused on the goal ahead, we rush through the transitions to get to the other side, even if the other side isn't any more important than the transition to it. We don't like stopping, changing, and being in-between. But if we can bring our attention to those moments of transition, acknowledging the impatience that may accompany them, we begin to feel more in our bodies, in the present moment, and more relaxed. The best way to bring our attention to the transitions—after remembering to do so—is to slow down. Just by slowing your hands you can relax and attend more easily. Slow down your hands while diapering and bathing your baby, and slow down as you move between poses in a sequence. Then notice what happens.

Did You Know ...

Baby-care books have been popular in the West for generations. Mostly written by men, they are reflections of both authorial bias and the particular social era in which the author lived. When Alison's grandmother was raising her children in the 1920s, the country was between two world wars, and science was ascendant. She kept baby diaries in which she described her babies' schedules and observed her children's behavior. In those diaries, you can hear the influences of the expert of the time, John Watson, a behaviorist who studied animals. He advised mothers to be scientifically minded and emotionally uninvolved. In Watson's opinion, mothers should adhere to specific schedules and ignore a baby's cries if it isn't time to feed. Babies were to be raised to be self-sufficient and self-reliant, and parents were taught to mold babies' behavior with the use of rewards and punishments.

It's painful for Alison to read her grandmother's diary entries, in which she writes, "I'm learning not to mind at all when Gigi cries when it isn't feeding time," and "Yesterday I didn't give in to my desire to pick up and cuddle Gigi. I don't want to ruin her."

Fast forward to the 1950s postwar America and Dr. Spock, who told mothers to throw out the scientific manuals and follow their own instincts. With the postwar economic boom and the increase in labor-saving devices in middle-class homes, women who weren't working outside the home suddenly had more free time than in any previous generation. That set the stage for on-demand feeding and the perception of happy mothers and babies with lots of leisure time.

With these changes came the child-centered home of the mid-twentieth century. Freud was becoming a household name, and his theories led to the belief that later development depended largely on how your mother treated you in infancy. Suddenly mothers were made to feel solely responsible not only for their babies' physical well-being but also for their future psychological health. Mothers were seen as the cause for any problem: a mother who was "smothering" caused her child's asthma; a mother who was distant was referred to as a "refrigerator" mother and was seen as the cause of her child's autism. Of course, we know now that these conditions are not caused by a mother's behavior.

The pendulum continued to swing in the child-manual literature. According to Ann Hulbert, in her book *Raising America: Experts, Parents, and a Century of Advice about Children,* every single prominent parenting "expert" from the twentieth century was either reacting against or trying to live up to his or her own parents, and then wove those subjective experiences into iron-clad, so-called scientific theories about what children need. Even Gina Ford, who is the queen of strict schedules, had a childhood that was chaotic and a mother who experienced mental health problems. It's interesting to note that Gina Ford slept with her mother until she was eleven years old.

There is such a diversity of information and contradictory advice that parents are left to pick and choose strategies that seem useful. It's no wonder that parents often pick a strategy that either meets their needs for healing from their own difficult childhood or emulates their happy one. When Alison looks back on her early years as a mother, she can see that many of her decisions and desires were a reaction to the insecurities she felt as a child. Some of the decisions were small, like putting sweaters on her toddlers when *she* was cold. But others were more complex, born of what she came to understand as her own—not her sons'—childhood struggles. As you seek out advice and information, be mindful of why one approach might resonate more with you. And, as always, practice self-compassion as you embark on the lifelong, entirely human, and entirely shared experience of differentiating *your* lived experience from your child's.

There's an App for That! (But It Might Not Help)

With mothers' increasingly busy schedules, there has been a rise in the popularity of apps as tools for new parents, helping them track and monitor their baby's growth, development, and schedules. There are apps developed specifically to help mothers reduce stress and find like-minded mothers nearby. If we add the rise of social media, parenting advice has definitely gone from the centralized expert-driven model to a peer-to-peer model of information gathering.

And if we look at other cultures, we can find much variation as well. Parents in many countries, including Spain, regularly put their children down after ten at night, because they believe it is important for the family to have time together in the evening after the busy day. In Egypt, family members sleep on a mattress for a fairly brief period during the night and then everyone takes a two-hour nap in the afternoon. Hunter-gatherers, like the Efe of Zaire, have no sleep schedules whatsoever; they stay awake till they are tired and then go to sleep.

There is no one rule book on sleep and feeding schedules. There is no scientific evidence that strict schedules or baby led schedules are better for a baby's development. But there is more than enough information and tools out there to help you find your sweet spot with your baby. Ultimately, though, you will find what works for you and for your baby by trial and error.

One Minute Yoga 7

GRACE 7

+ *Gather* yourself in child's pose and feel your belly move against your thighs as you breathe. Notice if you feel any tight muscles in your thighs or back and shoulders.

+ *Rest.* Gently roll your forehead on the matt to the right, then left, while you breath deeply.

+ *Ask* "Right now, where do I feel tight, where do I feel loose? Am I holding my breath or is my breath moving freely?"

+ *Compassionately* and kindly, send breath and awareness to those parts of you that feel too loose or too tight.

+ *Engage* again with your day, feeling not too tight and not too loose. Begin again.

Breathing 7

Three-part breathing with a short hold. Notice if there is any tightness when you inhale deeply. If so, slow down your inhale a little and soften your belly. Now pause at the top of the inhale and bottom of the exhale. How does it feel in the space at end of the inhale? Does it feel different in the space at the end of the exhale? Repeat three times.

Asana 7

PLANK

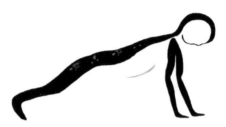

- ◆ Stand in mountain pose.

- ◆ Raise your arms up on your next inhale, exhale, and fold forward, with knees bent.

- ◆ Walk feet back until you are in a high pushup position. Your hands should be under your shoulders, fingers pressing into the floor. Pull your navel in toward your spine.

- ◆ Hold plank for three full breaths. It's okay to shake, and it's okay to drop down to your knees, rest, and then come back into plank.

- ◆ On the next inhale, lift your hips toward the sky into downward-facing dog, hold for one cycle of breath, feeling your heels leaning toward the floor.

- ◆ Walk your feet forward to meet your hands, bend your knees, engage your abdomen, and come up to standing in mountain pose.

FLOW

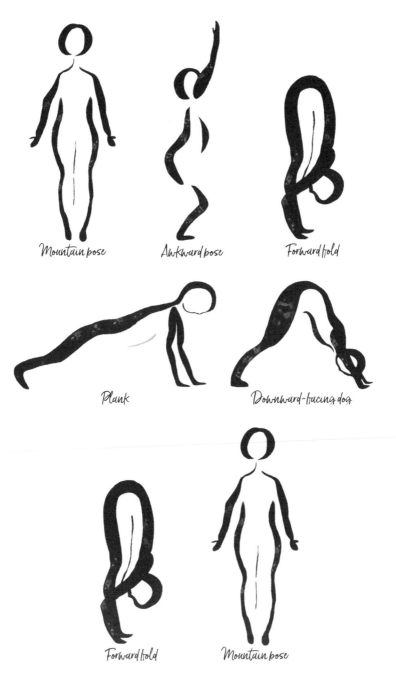

Mountain pose

Awkward pose

Forward fold

Plank

Downward-facing dog

Forward fold

Mountain pose

In a flow, we lead with our breath, and the movement follows. Notice, as you go through the flow, if you are tense or striving. Are you holding plank even after your wrists hurt? If so, just notice and drop your knees to the ground. Or are you feeling too loose? Notice and then pull your muscles in toward the centerline of your body. Pay special attention to the transitions between poses, whenever possible.

- Mountain pose—Come to standing and feel your feet solidly on the ground.

- Awkward pose—Bend your knees on an exhale, inhale, arms pointing up and forward, so your forearms are next to your ears.

- Forward fold—Exhale and sweep your arms down in front of you as you fold forward.

- Plank—Inhale and walk your feet toward the back of your mat, keep your spine straight and navel draws toward your spine. Hold plank for a few breaths.

- Downward-facing dog—Inhale and lift your hips toward the sky. Exhale.

- Forward fold—Inhale and walk your feet to hands. Hang out in forward fold, knees bent, if you like.

- Mountain pose—Inhale and engage core to come back to standing. Feel the effects of the flow.

You can do this flow three times or add this flow to the previous practice for a longer practice. Speed up the flow and then slow it down. Notice how different it feels.

Mantra 7: **Not too tight, not too loose.**

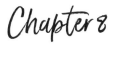

Chapter 8

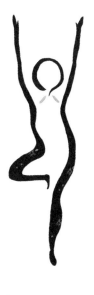

Tree Pose

Just as Maddie was slipping out the back door, she heard the doorbell ring. She cursed under her breath.

"Hey, Maddie, are you still here?" her husband called from upstairs. "Can you get the door? I think it's my parents. I keep telling them they don't have to ring the bell, but they keep not listening."

Maddie considered ignoring her husband, pretending she was too far out the door to hear him. But she didn't. "Got it," she called.

Maddie's in-laws were in town to help out with the baby because the nanny was sick. She opened the front door and greeted her in-laws with hugs and kisses and thanks, and she was just about to say she had to run out the door when another car pulled up in the driveway, causing Maddie to curse again, this time not entirely under her breath. She'd entirely forgotten that her husband's best friend was coming in from New York for a wedding, and they'd offered—no, *insisted*—that he stay with them instead of getting a hotel. "Come in, come in!" Maddie said. More kisses, more embraces, all around. All the while Maddie tried to stay as close to the front door as possible, hoping she could still make an inconspicuous exit.

"Mads?" Maddie's husband called down in a loud voice that seemed, to Maddie, to be at odds with his task, which was getting the baby to take a nap. He sounded frustrated. Maddie felt her heart sink. She put down her purse and keys. "Coming," she called back brusquely, then turned, smiling, to her houseguests. "Make yourselves at home!" she said, hoping her invitation sounded more genuine than it was.

Four months before Maddie had circled this very day on her calendar and written "Piano sale!" in bright red marker inside the day's box, a particularly noticeable announcement on an otherwise mostly empty calendar. Since becoming a mother, Maddie hadn't made many plans. This wasn't to say she had a lot of free time—she had no free time at all, in fact. She worked full-time and had an eight-month-old baby. Maddie knew there were a lot of things she should have on that calendar: date nights with her husband, that infant CPR class she kept meaning to take, Mommy-and-Me swim classes.

But there didn't seem to be time for those things. There wasn't really time for the piano sale either, but Maddie was determined to make time. Because if she didn't, she'd have to wait an entire year for the sale to happen again. She'd already been waiting for what felt like forever. Maddie had played the piano since she was six years old. She wasn't a star musician; she just loved to play and always had. All through her early life, whenever she had been worried or sad or trying to make a decision, she had always sat down at the piano. But since finishing college, she'd lived in a series of apartments on a series of small incomes, and she hadn't been able to have a piano. Now she was married, with a better job and a house, and it was time. Every time Maddie walked into her house, she saw the blank wall she'd saved for the piano.

"I can't figure out what's going on," Maddie's husband said to her as she came into the darkened nursery. He was bouncing around the room with the baby in his arms. The nap-time music was playing on the portable speaker, the room-darkening shades were drawn, and the lavender mist was billowing from the essential oil diffuser. It was so sleep-conducive that Maddie could barely keep herself from lying down on the floor. She blinked hard, trying to stay awake. "Your parents and Keith are downstairs."

Her husband looked confused. "Keith's here?"

"Yeah," Maddie said. "Remember how we invited him to stay?"

Her husband groaned. "Oh, crap, I totally forgot about that."

Maddie wanted to be annoyed, but she'd forgotten too. "Well, he's here, and so are your parents."

"Great," her husband said. "And this kid's not at all tired." The baby howled and lunged for Maddie. She stepped back a little.

"Maybe he's dropping his third nap," Maddie said, trying as hard as she could not to make eye contact with the baby.

"Already?" her husband asked.

"He's eight months old," she pointed out. "We're probably lucky it lasted this long. Listen, I have to run. It's the piano sale."

"Now?" her husband said. "But everyone's here."

Maddie felt terrible. "I know," she said, "but this is my chance."

"Well, can you take the baby with you? Keith was going to help me stain the deck."

Maddie shook her head. "I can't. It's going to be a madhouse."

"Can you go tomorrow?"

"It's one day," Maddie said, feeling impatient. "Once a year, remember?" She had a newly familiar feeling in her stomach, a feeling that she was going too far in one direction. Sometimes it was the direction of work, away from the baby, which felt crappy, and then sometimes it was the direction of the baby, away from pretty much everything else, and that felt crappy too. It was why she needed the piano. So that she could finally do something else, something that wasn't for the baby or work. Something that was just for her.

"I have to go," Maddie said, feeling terrible, but doing it anyway, hoping that someday, somehow, all of this was going to get easier.

~ ~ ~

> *To lose balance sometimes for love is part*
> *of living a balanced life.*
> —ELIZABETH GILBERT

~ ~ ~

A wise and honest mother Erin knows once said, "I love my baby more than life itself, but I still love life." We think this is an extraordinary statement, one that has the potential to expand women's lives in all stages of motherhood. And it is one of the many ways to begin answering the question that so often begins to arise in this time: How do we, as mothers, feed our personal *and* maternal passions, passions that seem to so often be in opposition to each other? Do we give things up? Do we carve out time for purely pleasurable experiences? For the things we create just for the sake of creating?

We're not talking about painting frescos or writing the great American novel here (unless one of those *is* your passion, in which case, we are behind you!). But for the most part, we're talking about more everyday creative acts and passions. Marathon running, banjo playing, political activism, knitting, surfing, meditation, movie watching, bulb planting, *New Yorker* reading. Taking pictures of flowers with your phone when you walk about the block. We're really just talking about that fundamental—yet easily forgotten—human experience of joy for joy's sake. And joy for joy's sake (or should we say joy for *your* sake) is something that can be elusive in the early years of motherhood.

So then, how do we do it? How do we allow ourselves the time and space for our passions? We start small. We think about the small movements and adjustments that keep us standing. And we stay away from drastic proclamations, from fatalistic narratives ("I'll never finish a project again, so why start?"). We also stay away from making rigid, ambitious schedules and plans that we can't help but abandon. And then we get creative. We seek temporary, imperfect solutions.

When Erin's first baby was around eight months old, all Erin wanted to do was read the *New Yorker*. She hadn't made it through a story since her baby was born. So Erin took the baby to the childcare center at the Y and then sat in the lounge section of the women's locker room and read for two hours. It was delicious. Of course she didn't get any exercise that day, and her daughter caught a cold in childcare. It wasn't something she would do everyday, but it was something she needed to do that day. It wasn't a perfect or permanent solution; it was a small motion in the direction of her passion. It was a reach.

A Moving Balance: A Shaky, Imperfect, Often Chaotic, and Always-Moving Balance

At the intersection of motherhood and our other interests, there is balance. Balance is never static. We don't achieve balance in motherhood once and for all. There is movement to balance. Like a tree, you have to continually move, making slight adjustments in response to your surroundings. Swaying is a sign of flexibility and strength. Fear of motion (and of falling) has a negative effect on balance, because we tend to tighten in reaction to fear, making it harder to sway and wobble. If we can see a fall—in yoga and in life—as both a consequence of *bold courage* and an *opportunity* to grow stronger, we will learn to wobble with grace.

When we practice balance in yoga, we actually create instability and asymmetry. This is also what Maddie did on the day of the piano sale, when she insisted on going despite the fact that it wasn't a good day for her family. She leaned in one direction; she swayed and wobbled.

Willing to Wobble

Alison had been a potter for years before she got pregnant with her first child, but after giving birth to her son, she barely had time to look at the wheel in the corner of her basement, much less throw pots on it. But she was still thinking of pots. She kept her subscription to *Ceramics Monthly,* drew designs, and dreamed of glaze combinations for years and years. When her boys were teenagers, she began to take her love of pottery seriously again and made room for clay in her life and the life of her family. Looking back, she wishes she had been willing to find the time much earlier, to risk the wobble. She knows how much pleasure pottery gave her. But she also understands how hard it can be to put something seemingly frivolous ahead of caring for our children. Baby steps. There's time.

Motherhood Is Less about a Perfect Balance and More about a Sustained Wobble

In yoga, we sway, we wobble, and we strengthen our vertical central core muscles to stay upright. We actually challenge gravity! We focus on a still point, called a *drishti,* to help steady ourselves in balancing poses. This is what we must also practice as mothers, so that we can have some of that life we still love, despite our overwhelming love for our babies. We have to create a little chaos, some instability. We have to let the dirty dishes sit there, disappoint people (including spouses, in-laws, and even our babies!), leave phone calls unreturned one more day, put off changing the crib sheet, delay registration for Music Together classes. We have to turn inward for a moment, strengthen that core that tells us what we want and who we are, and strike out in a new direction. And then we have to wobble, joyfully.

As we wobble, we remember that the goal isn't to stay perfectly balanced. The goal is to get comfortable with the wobbling and, yes, the falling. Sometimes we can't really know the feeling of balancing until we know what it feels like to fall out of balance, stand back up, and teeter some more.

If, at this point in motherhood, you have sacrificed large parts of yourself in order not to rock the boat, it might feel better to take tiny steps toward a different kind of balancing, experimenting with an hour alone—with your baby in someone else's care—so you can have some time to reflect. Or if you've gone back to work and become accustomed to time away from your baby so that you can do your job, but you can't imagine allowing yourself *more* time away to do something pleasurable, it's also good to start small, maybe with an extra thirty minutes of child-care so you can walk around the block. When you take that time, you can begin to ask yourself, *What is something that I love, something that I've sacrificed in order to keep life with my baby stable?*

By now you've been practicing self-awareness and self-kindness on and off the yoga mat, so we hope that, while the answers to this question might not come quickly, you'll begin to allow yourself the time and space you deserve to consider them. Accessing answers requires a certain kind of creativity. It requires more relaxed mulling rather than focusing, and it might be easier to conjure up the questions and then, instead of trying to answer them, just keep them in mind as you take a walk or go about your day and see what images and thoughts float around in your mind.

Some women like to draw or doodle and see what comes onto the paper. Keep with the questions until you begin to feel a sense, however murky, of what might be missing from your days with your baby. Then start to experiment with small (and imperfect!) ways to add those elements back into your life, knowing that you will feel torn, that you will fall in and out of balance. The more we practice and strengthen those balancing muscles, the easier it is to move between taking care of our child and taking time for our creativity and passions to flourish. The movement is made possible by an acceptance of ambivalence, which, as you remember from chapter 5, is a good thing. In other words, it's love that makes you wobble. Love on both sides.

Did You Know …

In yoga classes we are encouraged, while balancing in tree pose, to focus on a still point in front of us, a little above eye level. This is called *drishti* in Sanskrit. The practice of *drishti* develops concentration and stability. It steadies the mind, breath, and body. *Drishti* also means a larger point of view or clear seeing, like a bird's eye view or wide-angle lens. By concentrating our gaze and quieting our mind, we can see where we are headed in a way that frees us from a binary equation of "me or my baby," allowing us to instead see "me *and* my baby." That what is good for your baby is good for you, and what is good for you is good for your baby.

You can experiment with *drishti* in tree pose. Try the pose first without focusing on a still point and instead let your focus drift from right to left, up and down. Then try the pose while fixing your gaze on a still point. Notice if there is a difference.

Off the mat, when trying to balance your desire to pursue something that is meaningful to you with caring for your baby, think about taking a wider view, one that zooms out and looks at the situation from a distance. Steady your mind, calm your nervous system, and see if an answer comes more easily. Or take a walk and look off to the distance, to the top of a skyscraper or the ridge of a mountain, notice your breath, and wait for the answer. A mantra is like a verbal *drishti*, keeping us focused on something larger. Try saying "There is strength in wobbling." See if it rings true. If so, let it guide you in you decisions.

One Minute Yoga 8

GRACE 8

- *Gather* inward, in mountain pose, by finding something at eye level in front of you, one point to gaze at softly. Gather inward all the energy that you often spend outward. Gather it in with your breath, and bring your attention to your core. Feel your feet on the ground and the way your weight shifts from one part of your foot to another as you maintain your balance standing.

- *Rest* your jaw and shoulders. Notice your breath.

- *Ask* "Is there some important part of me that I have lost and that I want to reclaim?"
- *Compassionately* hold that part of yourself like you would a small baby, gently and with affection and curiosity.
- *Engage* with your day knowing you will fall in and out of balance. Begin again.

Breathing 8

Inhale to the count of three and at the top of the in-breath, sip in a little more air, just for you, as if sipping through a straw. Exhale with a nice long sigh. Repeat three times.

Asana 8

TREE POSE

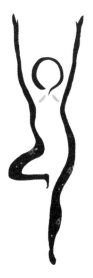

- Start in mountain pose.
- Find a spot at eye level in front of you to softly gaze at to help you balance. Your *drishti.*

+ Bring your hands to your hips or palms together at prayer in front of your heart.

+ Engage your core. Shift your weight to the left foot and bring your right foot to the inside of either your left thigh or your left ankle. Feel yourself wobble, maybe fall out of the pose (if so, steady yourself and try again), but notice the constant of your breath and continue to press your palms together or press your hands into your hips. Press your foot against your ankle or thigh, engaging your core, and lengthening your spine and crown toward the sky. Feel the strength along the center line of your body; there is stillness there even while you wobble. Gather your energy in toward yourself rather than out.

+ Repeat on the other side.

+ Shake out any tension in your feet and ankles.

+ If you have time, rest in *savasana* or child's pose.

(Note: You will find that you can balance easily one day and not at all the next. This is normal. So when you try tree pose, if this is a day when you find it impossible to balance on one foot, allow the foot against your ankle to touch the ground like a kickstand for more balance.)

Mantra 8: There is strength in wobbling.

Chapter 9

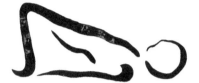

Bridge Pose

Jessie was doing the dishes when her phone lit up with a text. "Missed you at playgroup. Where were u?"

Jessie wiped her hands on a dish towel. "Molly napping," she wrote back. "Didn't want to wake her."

The reply was a thumbs-up emoji. And then, "Playground later?" with a cartwheel emoji.

Jessie hesitated before writing back. "I wish! In-laws for dinner. Have to cook."

A horrified-face emoji was the response, and then nothing.

Jessie put down her phone and turned to her baby, who was not, in fact, napping, but eating Cheerios in her high chair. Or, more accurately, throwing Cheerios onto the floor for the dog to eat. Jessie poured more cheerios onto the tray, then sat down at the kitchen table and cried a little. She hated lying to her friend about why she wasn't at playgroup, hated lying to all her other new mom friends when they asked her to go places with them or to come over for the morning and let the babies squabble over toys on the rug while they drank coffee on the couch and talked. Jessie hadn't actually gone anywhere with Molly in nearly a month.

A month before, Molly had gotten the flu. The real flu. The terrible, serious, dangerous-for-children-and-the-elderly flu. And this year's flu was particularly scary. There were stories about it on the radio and in the local paper. Jessie's pediatrician and the childcare center had sent emails urging parents to wash their hands and limit young children's exposure to crowds. Jessie followed all the precautions: she took Molly in for a flu shot, she washed her little hands after playgroup, she wiped down her toys.

But then, in early November, when Jessie's husband was away for work, the baby came down with a fever. It's just a fever, Jessie told herself. By then she'd gotten pretty good at fevers: give the baby a medicine dropper of Tylenol, put her in a cool bath, and give her a Popsicle, which, in itself, was pretty entertaining for both the baby and Jessie. But this fever was different. The baby was so fussy and was hotter than she'd been before. Jessie gave her Tylenol and called her sister.

"Try a Popsicle," her sister said. "And maybe put her in the bathtub?"

After what felt like an eternity, the baby finally fell asleep, on Jessie's chest. When Jessie woke the next morning, at six, it wasn't because the baby was crying; it was because the baby was so hot. Jessie reached for her phone. She called the pediatrician.

"Hold, please," the receptionist said when she answered.

"Hold, please," the nurse said when the receptionist transferred her to the nurse.

Jessie held.

"Kids First Pediatrics," the nurse said when she finally picked up after what felt like forever. "Child's date of birth?"

Jessie whispered her baby's birth date, not wanting to wake her.

"Excuse me?" the nurse said.

Jessie said it louder, the baby started to whimper. Jessie hated the nurse.

"How can I help?" the nurse asked.

"My daughter has a fever," Jessie said. "She's had it for two days."

"What's her temperature?"

"102," Jessie said. She hadn't actually taken the baby's temperature since she first got the fever, but she knew it hadn't gone down.

"And how long has she had it?"

"Two days," Jessie said.

The nurse asked her a few other questions, each one of them making Jessie more worried. Yes, she was coughing a little; yes, she was lethargic.

"Sounds like she has the flu," the nurse said.

"The actual flu?" Jessie said.

"Yes," the nurse said. "The actual flu."

"I'll bring her right in," Jessie said, starting to get up off the bed.

"Actually," the nurse said. "We ask that parents not bring children infected with the flu virus into the office. For the safety of our other patients."

The safety of other patients? Her baby was a danger to other kids? "Doesn't the doctor need to see her?" Jessie asked. "What about Tamiflu?"

"If she's had the fever for two days, then it's too late for Tamiflu to be effective," the nurse said. "There's nothing to do except push fluids and Tylenol, and let her rest. You can go right to the ER if she gets worse."

Jessie felt herself go cold. "What do you mean worse?"

"A temp of 103 or higher, trouble breathing, or a blue tinge to her lips or fingernails. That would mean she wasn't getting enough oxygen."

Jessie suddenly felt like she wasn't getting enough oxygen. "Can you tell me what comes before the blue lips?" Jessie asked. "I really don't want it to get that far."

"I think your daughter will be fine," the nurse said. "Just watch her carefully."

After she hung up with the nurse, Jessie started to cry. "I will never, ever take my eyes off you again," she said to her sleeping baby and to anyone or anything that was listening.

The nurse had been right. Molly was fine. Her fever broke; her lethargy ended. She healed. But Jessie was still suffering. She was terrified to take Molly out of the house, terrified that she would get another illness, something even more serious this time, and that she wouldn't be so lucky again. Jessie canceled her regular babysitter, stopped taking Molly to childcare at the gym, dropped out of music class, avoided playgroup. She didn't even take Molly to the grocery store. The whole world seemed so threatening, so entirely filled with danger. She didn't know how anyone—how any mother—could endure it.

~ ~ ~

> *I knew that if I allowed fear to overtake*
> *me, my journey was doomed. Fear, to a*
> *great extent, is born of a story we tell our-*
> *selves, and so I chose to tell myself a dif-*
> *ferent story from the one women are told.*
> *I decided I was safe. I was strong. I was*
> *brave. Nothing could vanquish me.*
>
> —CHERYL STRAYED

~ ~ ~

The stakes have never felt higher than when we become mothers caring for our babies. Sometimes we can put their terrible vulnerability out of our minds, but sooner or later, something happens. Life happens. An illness, an accident, a friend-of-a-friend's baby with a frightening diagnosis. Then we realize how little control we actually have. As mothers, we struggle with the fact of uncertainty. It's important to remember that you are not alone in this struggle. You share it with all mothers, throughout time, and across the world.

If you choose the path of resistance, like Jessie, you may have occasional and small wins, times when you manage to avoid an illness or accident. But for the most part, you will lose the war for safety in the face of the unknown. The more you try to prevent all the things that could go wrong, the less safe you will feel. This is because when you try to fight the dangerous unknown of the future, you are actually *practicing* worry. As your mind focuses on the details of potential tragic scenarios, you trigger and strengthen the stress response in your nervous system—fight, flight, or freeze. Jessie can't even take her baby to the playground for fear of the germs that might be lurking there.

Resistance to uncertainty and change can take many forms: perfectionism, over-involvement, and prevention rituals. Underlying uncertainty is the principle of impermanence. Everything is changing. Having a baby teaches us many things, and one is the constancy of change. Since you became pregnant, change has accelerated like never before, and this new rate can feel unsettling. The Buddha is said to have named impermanence—and our resistance to it—as one of the marks of existence that causes suffering. Of course, mothers don't need the Buddha to teach them about impermanence, they have a little Buddha in their arms every day. So how do we make peace with all this change and uncertainty about the future?

Baby-Proof Your Mind …

The first step, before you do anything else or make any plans for the future, is to decide what you can do to keep your child safe in this very moment, at this very stage. There are many practical things a mother can do to make her nine-month-old safe. These tasks and precautions are essential to your confidence and well-being, *and* your baby's safety, and we wholeheartedly encourage you to do them. But once you've bought the baby gates, installed the cabinet latches and electric-outlet covers, and put the glass coffee table in the attic, well, we encourage you to call it good.

So we say, do everything you can, by all means. And then stop and rest. Stop, rest, and, with some loving curiosity, take a look at your worry. Ask yourself, is all well right now?

The writer Courtney Martin explores the particular kind of anxiety that plagues mothers. She writes, "I am learning that to be a mother is to know that you can't know everything will be okay and still operate as if you could. The alternative is to have your entire body—heart, mind, and soul—be held hostage by fear. So I'm riding the waves of the oceanic anxiety that is motherhood—at least for me."

Oceanic anxiety. We love that image. Because it's so true: our anxiety is vast—so vast as to seem borderless—and highly responsive to the prevailing winds of internet stories, the changing tides of complex recommendations, of troubling new research. We also love it because, like children at the beach just learning how a boogie board works, we can learn to ride those waves. We can stay above the depths. We can recognize our own triggering riptides and move into other, calmer currents.

We can also move in the currents of our own life, not our baby's. Often, when mothers worry endlessly about their children, they aren't giving themselves—and their own feelings—the space they need. When Erin's first daughter was nine months old, she took her to Florida to meet Erin's grandmother. There were so many things to worry about: baby-proofing her grandmother's house, wiping down the rental car seat with antibacterial wipes, applying the right kind of sunscreen, getting the right kind of water wings. So many things, in fact, that Erin didn't have the mental space she needed to be present with her grandmother. Her anxiety over what might happen kept her from noticing and engaging with what was actually happening.

… But Don't Worry about Your Worrying!

The kind of fear or anxiety that Courtney Martin alludes to has, throughout history, been viewed as a pathology or psychological disorder of the individual rather than an existential truth of parenting. The truth is that, as mothers, we love our babies more passionately and more deeply than we could ever have imagined. We also can't, with any certainty, know our babies' futures. We can't know if they will be safe and healthy for the rest of their lives. And yet we keep loving them, keep investing in their health and safety.

This deep, ferocious love and the truth of uncertainty and mortality is the origin of mother fear, the kind of fear only a mother feels when she perceives danger for her child. Resisting the truth of uncertainty and the accompanying anxiety is the source of pain. If we can normalize and contextualize this truth, our vulnerability can become a badge of honor. Our courage can be our sign of belonging in the community of all mothers. We love in spite of the uncertainty; we invest completely, not knowing how it will turn out.

That is true courage.

As Brené Brown says, "Vulnerability sounds like truth and feels like courage. Truth and courage aren't always comfortable, but they're never weakness." And as the Buddhist poet Alan Watts wrote, "The only way to make sense out of change is to plunge into it, move with it, and join the dance."

But how can we "join the dance" and stop resisting?

Strong Back, Soft Front

First, we can acknowledge that our vulnerability is pretty unavoidable. You are already courageous beyond measure to love your baby so deeply in the face of uncertainty and change. Recognizing this fact, and allowing yourself to feel proud of your bravery, can help you to foster kindness toward yourself and to begin opening the door to uncertainty, knowing that you can handle it. You are already doing the hardest part.

Then, take a minute and recognize that every other mother you know is somewhere on the same path to befriending uncertainty and the anxiety that goes with it. You aren't alone. Why not talk about it? Our hope for Jessie is that she'll be able to share her worry and fear with her mother friends and that they'll be able to join her in her uncertainty, because the truth is they're already there, whether they want to acknowledge it or not.

The reality is that the uncertain future doesn't equal catastrophes, it really only represents the unknown. Thinking about all the catastrophic things that could happen in the future doesn't stop them from happening; it just feels like it will. The only thing it actually does is make us more anxious. So when you find yourself once again imagining a future filled with danger, it is possible and helpful to gently and kindly shift your attention to the present moment. Mindfulness of the present and anxiety about the future are incompatible. Another powerful antidote is to visualize things working out well. If you are going to have a movie of the future playing in your head, why not pick one that ends well. It's much more soothing.

The physical practice of yoga can embody (bring to mind through our body) a sense of groundedness, openness, and vulnerability with strength and courage. It brings our attention to the present moment, our breath, and movement, and is therefore soothing. We save bridge pose for the end of practice so our body is warmed up and our muscles are strong enough to support the opening of bridge pose without injury. There is a saying in Zen—"strong back, soft front"—that refers to the strength of our spine, which is the source of our integrity and our commitment. The soft belly is vulnerability, kindness, and compassion. In bridge pose, you can feel the opening of the front of your body while simultaneously feeling the strength of your back.

Tonglen for Motherfear

The practice we learned earlier in the book to help us cope with persistent crying can also help with moments of deep uncertainty. As an alternative to resisting uncertainty and fear—and all the coping mechanisms we adopt to keep it at bay—we can practice *tonglen*. When you start to feel the crush of anxiety descend, open your heart, breathe in the uncertainty, and breath out peace in this present moment. Ask yourself, is my baby safe right now? Breathe in the anxiety. Am I safe right now? If the answer is yes, breathe that out. Right now my baby and I are just fine. All is well right now. Breathe in anxiety, breathe out "we are just fine."

One Minute Yoga 9

GRACE 9

- ♦ *Gather* yourself by lying down on your strong back, knees bent, feet flat on the floor. Feel your back touching the floor. Feel the solid ground as a support. Feel held.

- ♦ *Rest* and soften your back muscles into the floor and follow your breath, without trying to change it.

- ♦ *Ask* "Am I safe right now? Is my baby safe right now?" Allow yourself to absorb the answer. Feel the sense of relief and safety in your body.

- ♦ *Compassionately* allow for any worried thoughts that arise.

- ♦ *Engage* with your day, feeling more secure in this moment. Begin again.

Breathing 9

Trusting your breath. Simply follow the breath with attention. Don't try to change or control it at all. Notice how, without any effort, your breath is always there, even if you seem to have forgotten about it. Simply bring your attention to your breath, as if coming back to a trusted home.

Asana 9

BRIDGE POSE

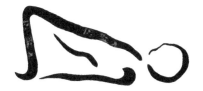

- Lie on your back.

- Bend your knees and bring your heels close to your hips. Arms by your sides, palms pressing into the ground.

- Initiate pelvic tilting by pressing your lower back and navel down to the floor while your tailbone lifts slightly. Bring your tailbone down and let the small of your back hollow. Repeat a few times to warm up your spine. Coordinate your breath and pelvic tilts in a comfortable slow rhythm.

- On the next inhale, slowly raise your hips toward the sky. Press the big toes down into the ground.

- Bring your chest toward your chin, feel the strength in your thighs and lower back and the openness of the front of your body. Strength and vulnerability at the same time.

- Exhale, lower your spine back to the ground while lengthening your spine, hips toward heels.

- Rest for a few breaths. Repeat.

HAPPY BABY: JUST FOR FUN

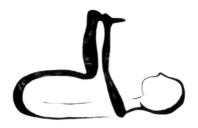

Happy baby pose reminds us that, like our baby, we can have moments to be present, undistracted by our anxious thoughts and enjoy the physical sensations of gently opening our hips and rocking back and forth. Feel free to play around.

- Still lying on your back, bring your knees up to your chest.

- Reach your hands toward the arches of your feet, ankles, or calves, and let your hips open

- Rock back and forth on your sacrum, and let your breath follow the rhythm of your movements. Allow yourself to be absorbed in the moment.

- When you feel complete, bring your knees together at your chest, wrap your arms around your shins and give yourself a big hug to prepare for *savasana.*

Mantra 9: Right Now, All Is Well.

Chapter 10

Savasana

It is impossible for you to go on as you were before, so you must go on as you never have.

—CHERYL STRAYED

You did it. You have taken care of your baby outside your body for as long as you cared for her inside. And now both of you are fully here, together *and* separate. You are two human beings engaged in the mother-child relationship. And you are also a woman engaged in her own unique experience of life with a child, knowing now that this life has it all: joy, chaos, pleasure, annoyance, satisfaction, boredom, and deep, deep love.

Now it's time for you to rest. To really rest. Even if it's only for a moment! Because now you know that a moment of rest can change everything.

As you rest, this is what we hope for you:

We hope you allow yourself to pause and re-center as often as you like, to return to yourself by tuning in to your body, breath, heart, and mind.

We hope you allow yourself to be kind—to yourself and to your baby—in easy pose.

We hope you allow yourself to be free of blame for your child's crying, sleeplessness, tantrums, and inability to share the shovels at the playground. We hope you give yourself the gift of warming up to new experiences and developmental phases; we hope you allow yourself to take child's pose whenever you need it. And to enjoy the sensual pleasure of a slow cat/cow whenever you feel stiff.

We hope you move forward in your own time, when you feel ready, and that you take breaks from Instagram and the doctored images of motherhood. We hope you keep in mind that important decisions take time. Becoming aware of your feelings and motivations takes stillness and time. We hope you can give yourself some breathing space and the permission to "not know, yet."

We hope you can give yourself permission to feel ambivalent forever, without the goal of resolution. We hope you remember that ambivalence is about having love on both sides. And we hope you continue to discover what's important to you so that you can stand strong in mountain pose.

We hope you give yourself permission to ease up when things get strenuous and then return—softer, stronger, and more resilient—to the awkward poses of motherhood.

We hope you give yourself permission to experiment with schedules and routines, to find freedom in structure, and to improvise until you find your flow, not too tight and not too loose.

We hope you give yourself permission to love your baby *and* your life, and to forsake the pressure of balance for the grace of wobbling in tree pose.

We hope you give yourself permission to open your heart and live your life in the face of uncertainty, the same uncertainty that all mothers experience, and to know that you are not alone in your worries. We hope you can remember that right now, all is well, and you can soften your guard because of your own strength in bridge pose.

And, most of all, we hope you can give yourself permission to rest. To pause, restore, integrate, and applaud yourself for all the ways you have navigated these months of motherhood with love and grace.

Savasana

It's time to do nothing in *savasana*. Just let your body melt into the bed or floor, follow your breath, and maybe whisper "I did it" on each exhale a few times. Some women find it helps to inhale and hold the breath while you contract muscles, and then exhale with an audible sigh and relax your muscles, just melting into the floor. Without doing anything at all, your nervous system integrates your practice as you surrender to gravity and melt. In the same way that your body breathes on its own, when you are resting, your body is integrating all the practices that have come before. Let go and do nothing for a few minutes, as often as you can.

The Ten-Minute Practice

We have combined all One Minute Yoga asana practices into a short but full practice. By all means play around with them. Improvise! Do what feels good when it feels good. Sometimes all ten practices will be the right amount of yoga, and sometimes you'll just want child's pose. Or tree pose. Or mountain. You'll do what feels right, and good. And then you'll get back to the raucous and complicated and mundane business of motherhood.

Remember: there's no rush. It's all waiting for you.

~~~

We have illustrated the full practice here, and an audio guide can be found at http://breathingspacefornewmothers.com.

Illustrated Practice

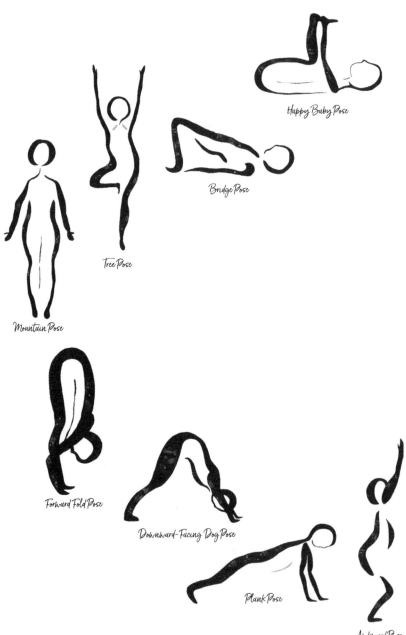

Happy Baby Pose

Bridge Pose

Tree Pose

Mountain Pose

Forward Fold Pose

Downward-Facing Dog Pose

Plank Pose

Awkward Pose

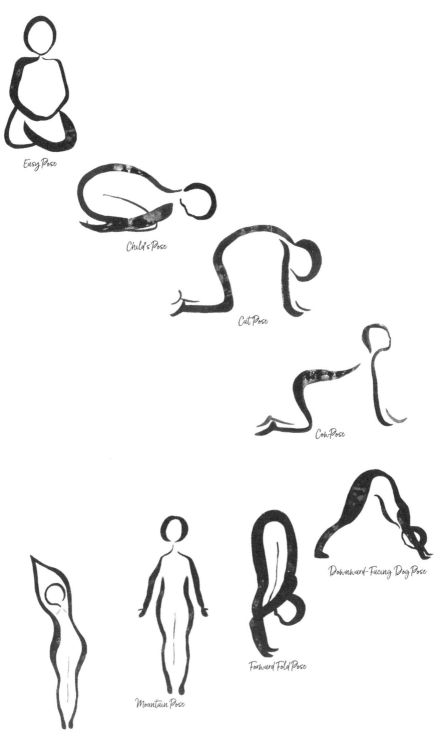

Easy Pose

Child's Pose

Cat Pose

Cow Pose

Downward-Facing Dog Pose

Crescent Moon Pose

Mountain Pose

Forward Fold Pose

Acknowledgments

This book grew out of a long career working with young families. There are so many people who have inspired, mentored, and informed my work. I wish I could name every single one of you individually.

Thank you to all the mothers I have had the gift of knowing: friends who are mothers, wise elder mothers, clients, and students. Especially, all the courageous young mothers who came to the Yoga of Parenting workshops. You asked for a book that could guide your daily practice at home. I hope *Breathing Space* will be that guide.

Alison Knowles trusted our vision and gave us a wide berth as she stewarded our project at North Atlantic Books. Gratitude to Yutaka Ai http://yutakaartofhealing.com for the illustrations; Ai paints with the intention of healing.

Thank you to the women who read early drafts, encouraged us, and gave insightful comments: Kate Nicholson, Lindsey Sterling Krank, Natalie Baumgartner, Sandy Hockenbury, and Nancy Sloane, among others.

My yoga and meditation practice is central to my life, my work, and this book. My many teachers have shaped my practice. Thanks to Jovinna Chan and Randal Williams, who taught my yoga teacher training at Kripalu Center for Yoga and Health. Randal and Jovinna are not only highly skilled in anatomy and alignment, but, more importantly, they also see the unique strengths within each student and enlarge on and mirror those strengths back, and in doing so, cultivate joy in moving meditation. I will be forever grateful to them and to Kripalu, a home for my practice of yoga, as well as a home for the best yoga teachers in the country. Boulder is filled with gifted yoga teachers, many of them mothers, too. I am grateful beyond description to practice with Nafisa Ramos, Steph Schwartz, Matt Kapinus, Kate Mulheron, and the rest of the crew at The Yoga Pod. You all kept me limber, lighter, and more present as I wrote this book.

I am indebted to Kristin Neff, who has defined and studied the concept of self-compassion and its effects on emotional resilience. It's been a game changer.

My point of view regarding mothers and small children grew out of my work in cross-cultural development and anthropology with Carolyn Edwards and Lella Gandini at the University of Massachusetts, Amherst. Because of them, I never made the mistake of thinking there was only one right way to raise a child or a mother.

Sylvia Boorstein's books and weekly talks have been an anchor for my practice and my teaching for the past fifteen years. Through her storytelling, she makes Buddhism accessible, meaningful, and funny.

To my daughters-in-law, two of the most loving and wonderful young mothers I know, thank you. I am blessed to have you in my life. I am learning about love and commitment from you both every day as you mother my delightful granddaughters.

Lastly, I still can't believe how lucky I am to have met Erin White years ago and then to have the opportunity to write this book with her. She is a dear and brilliant friend who often makes me laugh till I cry. Erin writes with clarity, subtlety, and heart, and, without her, this book would still be a bunch of coffee-stained file folders filled with some good ideas.

—AR

Thank you to the women who helped me become a mother. Ginny Miller was a gifted and generous midwife, and I still have her cellphone number taped inside my kitchen cabinet. My sister, Rebecca White, cared for me and my babies with love and tenderness, and continues to do so, all these years later. I met Patsy Kauffman-Barber in a prenatal yoga class fifteen years ago, and she instantly became my mother-comrade—a steadfast companion in the love, boredom, uncertainty, and hilarity of it all. Anne Truitt, Grace Paley, Rachel Cusk, Anne Enright, and Deborah Garrison wrote narratives of motherhood that saved my life, and my mind. I can't thank them enough.

Thank you to Stacey Mackowiak for Saturday morning yoga and friendship.

Thanks to Heather Abel for absolutely everything—in particular, for early help with the manuscript and for daily help with motherhood.

My deepest thanks go to Alison Rogers, for gifts of friendship, wise counsel, and delectable apricot jam. It was a delight to write this book with her, to have the chance for extended phone calls and visits, long hikes and swims and delicious dinners to clear our heads and send our conversations in new directions. I'm thrilled to see Alison's vision alive and in print, so that other women can know her as an honest, brilliant, and kind teacher and yogi. If only you could taste her jam.

—EOW

.

About the Authors

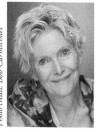

ALISON ROGERS earned a master's degree in counseling psychology from Harvard and a doctoral degree in dhild development from the University of Massachusetts, Amherst. After more than thirty years of clinical work as a therapist and educator, she trained as a yoga instructor at Kripalu and shifted her focus to create the Yoga of Parenting, a practice and philosophy that integrates principles from cutting-edge psychology with mindful yoga. Rogers has three grown sons and three granddaughters and lives in Boulder, Colorado.

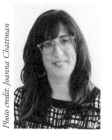

ERIN O. WHITE'S work has appeared in the *New York Times, Creative Nonfiction, Portland Magazine, On Being,* and elsewhere, including several anthologies. She is the author of *Given Up for You: A Memoir of Love, Belonging, and Belief.* She lives in Minneapolis with her wife and two daughters. For more about her work, visit http://www .erinwhite.net/.

About North Atlantic Books

North Atlantic Books (NAB) is an independent, nonprofit publisher committed to a bold exploration of the relationships between mind, body, spirit, and nature. Founded in 1974, NAB aims to nurture a holistic view of the arts, sciences, humanities, and healing. To make a donation or to learn more about our books, authors, events, and newsletter, please visit www.northatlanticbooks.com.

North Atlantic Books is the publishing arm of the Society for the Study of Native Arts and Sciences, a 501(c)(3) nonprofit educational organization that promotes cross-cultural perspectives linking scientific, social, and artistic fields. To learn how you can support us, please visit our website.